Recoveries

True Stories by People Who Conquered Addictions and Compulsions

*****

edited by
Lindsey Hall & Leigh Cohn

Gürze Books

Recoveries

True Stories by People Who Conquered Addictions and Compulsions

Gürze Books
P.O. Box 2238
Carlsbad, CA 92008
(619) 434-7533

Library of Congress Cataloging-in-Publication Data

Recoveries: true stories by people who conquered addictions and compulsions.

Bibliography: p.

1. Compulsive behavior--United States--Case studies.
2. Substance abuse--Patients--United States--Biography.
3. Eating disorders--Patients--United States--Biography.

I. Hall, Lindsey, 1949- II. Cohn, Leigh

RC533.R43 1987 616.86'0092'2 87-19810

ISBN 0-930677-11-5 (softcover)
ISBN 0-930677-12-3 (hardcover)

First Edition

10 9 8 7 6 5 4 3 2 1

"Chronic remorse, as all the moralists are agreed, is a most undesirable sentiment. If you have behaved badly, repent, make what amends you can and address yourself to the task of behaving better next time. On no account brood over your wrongdoing. Rolling in the muck is not the best way of getting clean."

Aldous Huxley
Brave New World

Table of Contents

Introduction

by

Lindsey Hall and Leigh Cohn

***

These stories are as gripping as the best fiction, but they are entirely true. The expertise of these authors, who describe their own experiences here, comes from the darkest moments of personal despair and triumphant achievements through recovery. Their accounts will provide insight into the nature of addiction for professionals and lay persons alike, but they will be especially inspirational for those personally struggling with addiction or who are directly affected by someone who is addicted. Whether cross-addiction is an issue for the reader, as it was for several of the authors, or there is an interest in one specific area, each section can be helpful. Although they had different experiences with various compulsions, one important thread ties each of these individuals together—they all recovered from the disease of addiction.

These seven chapters are about ordinary people: mothers and fathers, sons and daughters, rich and poor, office workers, students, housewives, and doctors. None of them wanted to get addicted. Most of them drank, smoked, dieted, or used drugs with friends, as many people do. Surely, they did not expect these diversions to get so extreme. Outwardly, few of them seemed consumed with the pain and self-doubt that dominated their lives. No one could have guessed the extent to which Charlie McMordie was using drugs, not even other users. Friends did not realize that when they bought cocaine with him he was hoarding for himself, or that he went on private binges. Even his wife had no idea that his lies about drug use would eventually destroy their marriage. Another chapter author, Lindsey Hall, seemed perfectly normal. Over a nine year period, she studied, worked, was married, and had friends; but unknown to everyone, she secretly overate and vomited four or five times daily.

The writers of this book do not philosophize or present scientific data to explain the genetic, biomechanical, or psychological factors of addiction. Our purpose is not to analyze why one person is a social drinker while another is alcoholic or why so many people accept yo-yo dieting as a way of life while others become so obsessed by losing weight that they starve themselves to death.

What this book does offer is an invitation to compare, to relate, and to be inspired. Each story provides its own explanations for what contributed to that author's choice of self-destructive behavior. Each person was influenced by their culture and families, but their paths were also paved by momentum which caused their methods of escape to get beyond control. In every case, the addiction became the main concern and nothing else—including life itself—mattered as much until they chose to recover. Although the chapters address different types of addictions, readers will discover personally relevant ideas throughout, and might find in any one tale the impetus to motivate change. Unlike "self-help" books which provide answers for particular problems, and with them inherent risks of not correctly following the prescribed recovery program, this book offers a wide range of solutions that invites readers to identify and select what to apply in their own cases.

Actually, readers struggling with addiction—alcoholism, for example—may get as much insight to their obsessive drinking from the other chapters as they will from the alcoholism story. An alcoholic who uses drinking as a method of coping will be able to see that Hall used bulimia and McMordie used cocaine, alcohol, and other drugs in the same way. Moreover, some readers may think it would be hard to relate to the experiences of a middle-aged Indian who spent half of his life drunk and homeless on skid row. After all, Robert Sundance's story of chronic alcoholism certainly would appear to be more extreme than the lives of most people who might pick up this book. No one expects their drinking to lead to 20 years of sleeping in parking lots and being unable to get up in the morning without a bottle of cheap, rot-gut wine. Sundance clearly did not expect that fate, though it happened. Perhaps his descent from social drinker to society's gutter may be exactly what a problem drinker needs to read.

Our culture encourages obsession. Standards of beauty and prestige are based on fad and fashion, often to the exclusion of health and personal preference. When Diane DuCharme began smoking cigarettes, it was fashionable and considered glamorous to smoke. She did not consider the ill effects on her heart and lungs, that her hair and clothing stunk, or that she would eventually turn to a cigarette to complement every emotion, whether it be to escape from momentary pain or reward herself for a job well done. In the same way, McMordie tried to emulate counter-culture heroes during the drug revolution of the late 1960s and early 1970s, which in turn led him to dependence on cocaine. It was only in recovery that it became apparent to them that our culture is not necessarily a place to look for behavioral standards.

Moreover, besides selling images that perpetuate these myths, society abundantly provides the stuff of which addictions are made, and places a general emphasis on external methods of coping. We've been convinced to look for easy answers to life's complex problems. Had a hard day at the office? Unwind with a stiff drink or take a drug. The advertisements show that good friends drink beer and wine together, not that they get drunk every night and have abusive, self-centered relationships. Having trouble finding a man to love you? Lose weight! A woman who weighs more than a slinky magazine model can turn the page to find the latest diet that will provide her with happiness.

Unquestionably, life is filled with everyday pressures, and we all search for some kind of relief. However, the same activities or substances that provide escape become an addict's primary focus. Bob MacFarlane was a physician who used medication to numb the pain of his surgical patients, but he used the same drug to numb his own anxiety. It was not long before the stress from his own usage was far worse than any of the problems he was looking to alleviate. Compulsive dieters can only think of eating. Alcoholics need to drink. DuCharme could not make it through a single night's sleep without waking up in the darkness of her room to have another cigarette. Addiction becomes more important than health, work, friends, loved ones, or life itself.

The authors also discuss how their families contributed to their obsessions. Some had parents who were addicted, and most of the families—though not all—were dysfunctional. In the chapters, no one places the blame in their upbringing, but the influences are apparent in the narratives of the stories. Avis Rumney learned about relationships and coping in a home with an alcoholic father. Instead of turning to booze, however, she used anorexia nervosa. McMordie's father was also an addict, besides which, family oil and ranching money financed his expensive drug habit. All of the men in Sundance's family were heavy drinkers; and, Janet Jacobsen was influenced by her father's death to use suicide attempts as a way of getting attention and escape. These stories provide models of co-dependence, children of alcoholics, families of divorce, as well as growing up in "normal" homes and still becoming addicted. An important part of recovery for these authors was learning to take responsibility for their own lives, accepting their roots, and making peace with their pasts.

A powerful component of addiction is denial—not admitting that there is a problem. In a few of the stories, the authors wake up after passing out from substance abuse and cannot understand why their loved ones are concerned, angry, or embarrassed. Although obvious to anyone else, it was hard for the addict to see the truth. Practically all of the writers experienced deteriorating health but refused to draw a connection to their addiction. The bulimic failed to concede that her sore throats and extensive tooth decay could be caused by vomiting. The smoker merely accepted "hacker's cough" and bad breath. Infections from repeated narcotics injections almost resulted in amputation but did not propel the user to stop shooting up. Even the skid row drunk kept cleanly shaved while he waited to be discovered for a leading role in Hollywood movies. Not only did denial prevent them from recognizing their problems, but it also perpetuated the momentum which sank them into further despair.

One after another, these authors hit rock bottom before they could seek recovery. Several of them first turned to suicide as a cure. Without acknowledging that his drug use was the problem, McMordie thought a bullet through his skull would finally bring him rest. With his knowledge of the human body, Bob MacFarlane understood exactly what it would take to end his life. After taking five times the lethal dose of sleeping pills, he slipped into unconsciousness prepared for death and the ultimate solution to his narcotics habit. But, whether it was due to true love or divine intervention, he was saved—at least for a little while. For months, he was overwhelmed with shame and guilt, and he could not imagine ever returning to the insanity and degradation of being a junkie. He sought new ways of finding spiritual fulfillment, improved his health with a new diet and exercise regime, changed jobs and living environments, and married the woman who loved him. But, for all these efforts, he returned to drugs. All of the people in this book were absorbed in their own self-destructive roles, and none thought that they could go any further into despair. In that way, their personal accounts are identical and can be easily identified with by readers who find themselves out of control.

Perhaps the greatest message in this book is that even people who are lost beyond hope can conquer their demons. In many instances, intervention was necessary. It came in the form of professional help after being institutionalized against one's will, from the wisdom of a small child, or through the support of a loved one. Several of these authors experienced personal miracles which gave them courage to change their behavior. By "accidentally" seeing a magazine article, Lindsey Hall discovered that she was not the only person in the world who compulsively binged and vomited; and, fortunately, the article's author was a therapist who only lived a few miles away. Both Charlie McMordie and Janet Jacobsen describe signs from God that inspired them to break away the barriers to change.

For most people, recovery is a long process that includes being knocked down, getting up, and then being knocked down again and again before having the strength to stand. The recoveries in this book involved professional therapy, a commitment to getting better, following a plan of action, and rallying from setbacks. All of the authors found that there were other people who could help them, and the fellowship of recovery is an ongoing theme that is juxtaposed with the loneliness of addiction. An essential part of getting beyond obsessions is being open and honest with others. Some of these people remained in support groups years after the behavior ended. Even those who quit "cold turkey" after many years of compulsing needed support from loved ones. None of the authors suggest that their experiences can be used as a "how-to" cure, but the combined strength of all of their successes provides tremendous insight into what it takes to overcome any addiction.

Each of their ongoing recoveries includes continued service to others suffering as they once had. Some of them now work professionally as counselors and therapists in their areas of addiction. In addition to these chapters, several write about recovery in their fields. Many are involved with organizations devoted to increasing awareness and education on national and international levels. Some are promoting change through legal and legislative measures. And, one, Robert Sundance, has almost single-handedly led to wide-spread legal reforms in the treatment of public inebriates.

Ultimately, it was an innate desire to live instead of die that propelled them to find the strength to recover. As it happened, in every case the result of getting free from the compulsions also meant a happier, healthier, more meaningful existence. What is apparent in their writing, and is especially true in talking to them, is that now all of these individuals love themselves and their lives. They have honest relationships, are productive, and, without exception, they laugh a lot and enjoy living. They are determined never to again succumb to addiction.

Although these people are "ordinary," they are also uniquely special, which was only apparent once their addictions were conquered. It does not matter if someone is an alcoholic, cocaine addict, or obsessed with dieting: these compulsions prevent them from living. A junkie's despair is no worse than a bulimic's or a person who is suicidal. As long as they permit themselves to be governed by their addictions, they cannot find contentment. The authors in this book convincingly show that anyone can recover. Life is to be lived and loved, not to be avoided, and their stories prove that this is true.

ALCOHOLISM

About the Author

Robert Sundance's story proves that even someone who is "on the lowest rung of society's totem pole" can change "the system." Drunk, homeless, and living on skid row for more than 20 years, 200 times with the D.T.'s, arrested 500 times and denied his legal rights, Sundance was determined to be heard in court. Over a ten year period, he spent an average of 226 days in jail each year waiting to plead his case. He believed that his jailings for public drunkenness were cruel and unconstitutional, because his alcoholism was a disease.

There are many ways his life could have ended. Alcohol could have killed him, like his drinking friends who died from cirrhosis of the liver before the age of thirty. He might have had a heart attack from the D.T.'s while left unattended in the drunk tank like others he knew, who were cremated under false names. The elements could have finished him off while he slept in skid row parking lots, blanketed by nothing more than the cheap wine in his body.

Robert Sundance lived to fight and win. His landmark court case drastically reformed the process of arrest and treatment of public inebriates. In Los Angeles County, where the *Sundance Decision* was won, these arrests dropped from more than 50,000 to about 1,000 per year. He beat alcohol, has been sober for twelve years, and is Executive Director of the Indian Alcoholism Commission of California. His victories show that regardless of the depths of addiction, individuals can be healthy, productive, and have meaningful lives in recovery.

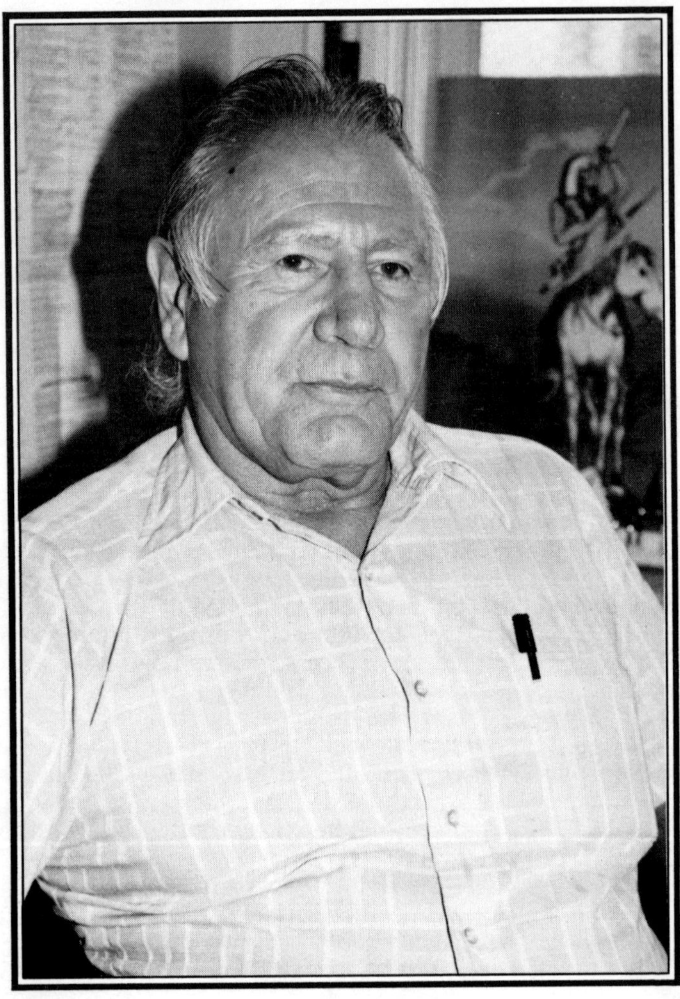

Robert Sundance

Not Guilty on Skid Row

by

Robert Sundance with Leigh Cohn

***

Drinking: A Way of Life

I was born in 1927 on a Sioux Indian reservation in Wakpala, South Dakota. It's just a little town. There was unspeakable poverty, no jobs on the reservation—even to this day there's 90% unemployment on my reservation. I had four sisters and three brothers, and, fortunately, none of the girls drank, nor did my mother. But all of the men, my brothers and my dad, were heavy drinkers. On my father's side of the family they all drank.

I took my first drink when I was three years old. It was during Prohibition, although there actually was prohibition for American Indians from 1832 to 1953. For 121 years, there was nowhere in Indian America to buy alcohol. Indian leaders themselves insisted on that law because they were afraid that Indians would drink themselves to death. Other races that came to North America had been exposed to alcohol before, but when it was introduced to Indians it was new and the leaders sensed early the destructive effects that alcohol could have on the race.

My Dad made homemade beer. He had it behind the wood stove. It was terribly cold up there, and it was a big chore to keep the wood chopped and the stove burning. There would be raging storms for days and you couldn't see anything but blinding snow. My Dad stayed up for three days and nights brewing the beer and keeping the flame alive in the wood stove. Hidden behind the stove was a big crock, so no one saw me when I dipped my little tin cup into it and started drinking. It didn't taste good, but it sure made me feel good. It was pretty strong, and I got loaded as heck! I was sitting high up on a sack of potatoes and I fell off, hitting my eye on the corner of a chair. My eye swelled up and closed, but it didn't even hurt. From that time on, I knew that if I drank I wouldn't feel pain; otherwise, I would have been screaming and crying.

Drinking was a way of life in those years, and seeing was learning. With the extreme poverty and hopelessness on the reservation, it was boring. There was no entertainment, so if you drank, you forgot for a while. It was an escape from reality.

I was getting drunk way before my teens, and then really boozed in my teens. My brothers and all the guys were drinking. It was a big thing on the reservation. I'd drink whiskey if possible, but it cost so much that we'd mostly drink home-brew raisin wine or beer. I used to know how to make home-brew out of anything. The main thing you had to get was sugar. Different guys would steal sugar from their homes and bring it to me for brew. I'd put anything into it: raisins, potatoes, rice, apricots, whatever I could get my hands on; and, God, that stuff came out strong. I think it was probably about 190 proof alcohol! It would really load you.

When I was fourteen, I used to go off the reservation to buy bottles because I looked older and White. Those guys who owned the liquor stores must have known that I was very young but they wanted the money and would sell it to me. I could buy whiskey or anything.

We used to drink fast because it was against the law and we had to get rid of the bottle. If we got caught drinking, the authorities would take the bottle away, so once it was opened, we'd throw away the cap and drink it down. Naturally, anyone would get drunk chugging a pint or a quart of whiskey.

I never believed I'd be an alcoholic or that I was doing anything that might hurt me. Even when I was just thirteen and fourteen years old, I'd have blackouts and remember nothing. No one told us that blackouts were from drinking too much or that there was anything wrong with that. I don't even think anyone around me knew that drinking caused problems.

I went to school on the reservation until eighth grade. In those days, higher education was not encouraged, especially for Indians. The system was run by Whites who discouraged Indians from getting a good education. I suppose they feared that educated Indians might take their jobs. The only jobs available to us were working for farmers who leased land on or near the reservation. That was hard work, sixteen hours per day, and we were only paid one dollar for a day's work, plus board and room. Those people would work you to death, but there was no other choice of work.

Drinking was already a way of life then, and all day I'd think about how much whiskey I'd be able to buy. All of my money went to buying booze, even though it was sometimes pretty hard to get in those days. All the guys who were worth anything—the best athletes, the rodeo riders, all of my role models—were drinkers and I wanted to be just like them. Hold your booze and drink all you can—that's how I thought life was supposed to be. I wanted to be a heavy drinker. I looked up to these people as heroes, but did not see that these terrific athletes would be burned out from drinking by the time they were out of high school. Even today, 71% of high school students, male and female, drink alcohol. That's why great Indian athletes don't excel into big time sports.

Military Service

World War II came along, and I wanted to get away from the reservation. There was nothing there, no jobs, extreme poverty, and I figured anything would be better than staying. I got a phoney birth certificate saying that I was seventeen years old and the military didn't care. They needed cannon fodder and took everybody. When I went into the Navy in 1942, I went in by myself. Most of my friends were going into the Army, but I thought it would be easier to get into the Navy because they were taking younger kids. I was lying about my age, and I think a lot of Indians did that, too. Actually, Indians are really patriotic. I wanted to serve a hitch in the Navy, then go into each branch of the service.

I especially wanted to enlist because I heard you could buy all the booze you wanted when you were in the service. You could just go to bars and buy all you wanted. I had money, and so did my friends. I wasted my liberties and everything because I was drunk all the time. I was a drunken sailor, a drunken Indian. That's the way I thought it was supposed to be. I tried to live up to that image.

They sent me to the Southwest Pacific, fighting the Japanese. I was a gunner on an aircraft carrier. You could deal with people in the medical department, who got 190 proof alcohol that the doctors used in the hospital. We'd cut it with grapefruit juice. Some pilots would come in from Australia and sell bottles of whiskey. They'd charge $50 to $100 for a bottle, but some of the guys would still buy it—especially the ones who were rich from gambling. Every chance I'd get, I'd drink. I couldn't drink every day, because booze was hard to get. That's why I didn't think of myself as an alcoholic.

When the war ended, I was honorably discharged and went back to the reservation. It was the same: unemployment, alcoholism, and nothing to do. A friend said to me, "Let's go back into the service, there's nothing here and at least in the service we'll have some money, board and room, and plenty of booze." He was going in the Air Force, so I left the reservation and went in with him.

Everything went well. I was drunk everyday, and worked in a warehouse issuing clothing. Alcoholics are smart, and I had a good memory—I still have a good memory, even after all the drinking. I could get drunk, especially on payday, but I was the only one who knew where everything was, so they wouldn't get rid of me. I was protecting myself and my drinking that way.

During my military career, I wouldn't go down to any skid row with my buddies, because I didn't want to be around all those winos and drunks. I didn't want to be like them, and I didn't think I ever would be. I didn't know that I was a drunk at the time, and if anyone had confronted me about it, I just would have denied it.

Then, alcoholics were not chastised in the service; but, just before the Korean War, a policy change came, and they started kicking alcoholics out. In 1950, I had a discharge hearing for chronic alcoholism. I didn't even know what the word "chronic" meant. "Alcoholic" was bad, but calling me "chronic" had to be worse. At my discharge hearing, the officers looked over my record and said, "He's a chronic alcoholic." That sounded terrible to me. One said, "He's a pretty good guy when he's sober, but he's never sober." Then another said, "He's just a drunken Indian, like the rest of them. He's a congenital alcoholic." I didn't know what that word meant either, but I didn't want to be branded either. Then an officer said, "He's an incorrigible alcoholic." I was embarrassed and didn't want to hear any more, so I said, "Just give me the discharge and let me out of here." They kept on going, "He was in the Navy, and all those Navy guys are a bunch of drunken sailors." Someone added, "He has some Irish blood in him, too," which was true, one of my grandparents was Irish. Then he said, "That's even worse, he's got to go." The ironic part of it all was that I used to see those same officers drinking all the time, too; yet, they threw around all those stereotypes about Indians, sailors, and the Irish. They finally gave me a dishonorable discharge. They kicked me out without any money, not even a ticket home. I was stranded in Omaha, Nebraska and hitchhiked back to the reservation.

Again, there was nothing, and I had to find a way to get out. The service had seemed like the only option. It was a good way for educating yourself. It did a lot of guys good, and they came back to the reservation to make changes and help our people. I thought I'd try joining the Marines, but with the dishonorable discharge I couldn't get in. I couldn't even get a job because of it. The military called it willful misconduct. Their attitude was that you got drunk because you wanted to, not because you were addicted and had to drink, and that's wrong. Thirty years later, I petitioned the courts and had that dishonorable discharge expunged and changed to an honorable, but what good did it do me?

On the Road and the D.T.s

I was 22 years old, on the reservation, with no options. After being in the service, I had seen the world. I knew there was more to life than the reservation. Finally, I just took off. I started drifting. I took odd jobs, and the main focus was, "How much booze will I be able to drink tonight?" When I'd blackout, I figured someone was doping the drinks, or maybe it was because I hadn't eaten anything. Not until I went into recovery years later did I realize that it was the alcohol doing it to me. The denial was too strong. Alcoholics won't admit that drinking is a problem.

I went to Rapid City, South Dakota. In those days I was able to work and drink. Of course, most alcoholics are not on skid row; they're part of the work force, keeping the family together. I would work and drink, rent a place for $10 a month, or stay with friends. In the drinking world it's a big fraternity and somebody always has booze. I used to drink with one particular family of four sisters. They all drank themselves to death before they reached their thirties; each one died of cirrhosis of the liver. I stayed in Rapid City for two or three years doing day labor, working in warehouses or on farms. One time we built a golf course. I'd make $8 per day, which seemed pretty good in the 50s. I'd work all day, get paid, and drink all night without sleeping for a week.

Alcohol is deceiving because it makes you think you're something that you're not. I thought I'd accomplish something great, like maybe become a movie actor. I thought I was husky and strong, but really I was weaker than hell. From the time I got out of the Air Force until a year or so later, I lost sixty pounds. I was drunk every day. One time when I was 22 years old, I got on a scale and thought the scale was broken. I was 6'3" tall and only weighed 152 pounds, down from my usual weight of 212. It was the first time I got the D.T.s.

That was the worst, scariest experience. It went on for five days. I was trying to impress someone that I didn't drink. They were friends in Rapid City, and I was working for them out in the country. I had been drunk day and night for a year, and I stopped drinking to convince them that I wasn't an alcoholic. While sitting in the bunk house reading some magazines around one in the morning, I heard some girls calling me. I knew there were no girls around there, but I went outside to see who was calling. It was dark and there were two broads dancing out there stark nude. I took off to the main house and woke up my friends and told them what I had seen. I made them go look, but no one was there, just a couple of butane tanks. They said it must have been their police dog making noises, but I knew it wasn't any dog that I watched. All night things like that happened. The next day I was going to haul hay in the field. Pretty soon I heard voices of some girls calling me from a bale of hay. Then another would call from a different bale of hay. I got scared and started running across the field. I ran so fast, I could have broken an Olympic record! The bosses got in a car and followed me and asked why had I taken off running like that. I said, "Those damn bales are all talking to me. The girls I've been drinking with are inside of the hay talking to me."

They took me to the hospital. On the way, I looked at a cloud and saw a face that told me I would die from cancer of the brain. When we got to the hospital, I told the doctor what had happened. He asked me how long I had been drinking. I was trying to impress them, so I said I wasn't drinking—denial again. He said, "Oh, yes you have," and asked me for how long. I admitted that I'd been drinking for three months, but really it had been more than a year. He explained that I was going through detoxification and that was why I heard voices. I told him I was going to die that night from cancer of the brain. He laughed and wasn't even frightened for me. He bet me $100 that I wouldn't die that night. I made him promise to send the money to my friends, where I lived. I waited in an examination room, and one woman kept peeking at me from around a curtain. Another hid beneath the examination bed. A nurse came in and I told her that two women were in there, and she ran off thinking I was crazy.

After five days, I felt like never having another drink. I felt tremendous. Had I never taken another drink, my life would have been completely different. I might have stayed around there, maybe married, but I would not have accomplished anything as worthwhile as my success with the Sundance case or my work with the Indian Alcoholism Commission. I'm fatalistic about my life, but I did waste thirty or forty years before I finally accomplished something. The excruciating pain and catastrophic ordeals that I went through at least led to great changes in society and the system.

People in jail often get the D.T.s. I've had them about 200 times. It's hard to get them the first time, but it gets easier and easier. After about fifty or one hundred times, you only need to drink one or two days and be cut off before you get them. The D.T.s are really amazing. You can talk to dead people and can even touch them. I thought it was a real world, and it was kind of fun and fascinating for about two or three days because everything that's forbidden in normal life, especially sexuality, is acceptable. I would look at a blank wall and be able to see movies, seeming to remember every scene. After the first couple of days, though, the D.T.s are a living hell.

Then people started killing each other and it got scary. Everyone that I ever harmed was after me. People from whom I tried to take girlfriends were coming with their buddies to beat me up, and they had knives and guns. My heart almost stopped. A lot of guys do have heart attacks from exhaustion and fear with the D.T.s because they can't sleep. Some people commit suicide because they get so scared. In jail, the authorities would often tie people down so they wouldn't hurt themselves during the D.T.s. Your nose is always running, you can't eat—I was afraid my food was poisoned—and these spirits, or whatever they are, keep pestering. If I closed my eyes, they'd come after me with a knife, so I had to open my eyes and stay awake. There's a fever in the brain. But when the D.T.s ended, I felt great. All the toxins are flushed out, and the whole body gets purified. All of the senses are at the peak of alertness. Colors are intense, sounds come through crystal-clear, and food tastes more delicious than ever. Everything feels great, the best in this world.

In any case, after I came out of it that first time, I was drunk again in about three days. I went to a rodeo and everyone was drinking. I was so scared by the D.T.s that I didn't ever want to drink again, but the physical craving was too great. I was burning for a drink. Everybody had bottles, and I was just going to have a little bit. I kept drinking and finally just took off again on the road.

I must have quit drinking 3,000 times, but for an alcoholic, you can't quit unless someone intervenes and you get into a program. Of course, I didn't know that then, and there weren't many recovery programs around, anyway.

A Skid Row Drunk

I was out of touch with my family for years and years. From Rapid City, I went to Billings, Montana for a few years, drifted to Minneapolis, to Seattle. I was in Chicago. I had to follow the bottle, and if drinking friends moved on, I would, too. For ten years I drifted on skid rows throughout the country until June of 1960, when I took a freight train from Phoenix to Los Angeles, where I spent 16 more years on skid row. Freight trains were a good way to get anywhere, and in those days it was safe. I used to ride them with women and no one would bother us. I rode to Los Angeles with a girlfriend and one other guy. I had a horrible hangover and was drunk from peppermint schnapps. I was so sick and thirsty on that train that I practically died. I would have died riding through the desert if this other guy hadn't found a whole block of ice somewhere during a stop. It lasted all the way to Los Angeles and saved my life.

At that time, I saw women mainly as a "piece of ass," and I had lots of girlfriends. They kind of liked me, who knows why. I was drunk all the time, never had any money, and put them through a hell of a life. I wasn't abusive, but I didn't care about anybody or anything except getting a drink and getting laid. Alcohol helps make sexuality uninhibited. It gives a sense of false courage. Sex plays a big part in alcoholism, and getting laid becomes second only to booze. During all of my drinking career, I strived for pussy, feeling superhuman in my sexual prowess. The alcohol intensified all of those feelings. Now, programs have sexuality workshops as an important part of recovery, because it is common for recovering alcoholics to have relapses and drink again in order to build sexual confidence. Alcoholics mistake sex for love, but sobriety puts sex and alcohol into proper perspective.

When I was drinking, if I had a woman with me, guys would buy me drinks. Usually, they were scheming on the broad, and I knew that, so I liked having women around with me. A lot of them died from cirrhosis—I can think of about six who died that way. About two weeks after I got to Los Angeles, I was thrown in jail, and the woman I arrived with went back home. I never saw her again. I sometimes had great dreams of settling down and getting married, but getting thrown in jail all the time breaks up a lot of romances. I think the police purposely try to interfere with your life. Lots of times a group would be drinking in the street and the police would throw the men in jail and let the women go. Every city I was in had lots of women on skid row living just like me.

By 1960, I was homeless and living in Los Angeles. I stayed there because it's really hard to get away from a place once you're there. You say, "Oh, I'm going to get off skid row, I'm going to get a good place to live, I'm going to get sober." I remember early on hearing one guy saying that he'd been on skid row for nineteen years and I thought, "Nineteen years! I would never stay on skid row for nineteen years." But I was drunk for over 30 years, and I drank on skid row in Los Angeles for sixteen years! I never dreamed I would be there that long. I thought I'd move back to Montana, or I'd go to Seattle, Portland, or Santa Barbara. But I couldn't even get out of downtown. In all those years, I never even saw the ocean. You can't get away. I wouldn't ride the bus because even thirty cents was a lot of money to me; a dime was a lot to spend on a phone call. I needed every penny to buy booze.

I used to be able to get up in the morning and work all day before getting drunk at night. Sometimes, I'd be too sick to work, and only worked a few days during the week. As the years went by, I got sicker and sicker and worked less and less. I'd wake up so damn sick, I'd have to drink at least a quart of wine just to get straight enough to get up. Whiskey is too strong. Wine is the only thing that'll calm the nerves and make you feel better. If I was trying to go to work, wine was the best thing to get me going. Then I could go to work and get paid, so I could drink more that evening. If I could get a few drinks during the day, that would help, too. Often, I couldn't work the whole day because I'd get too sick with no booze around. Fresh air practically killed me because I was so used to stale, downtown air.

Pretty soon you can't even work. That's when you get to be a hardcore skid row alcoholic. That's what happened to me in Los Angeles. It was better to be there than in one of the East or Midwest cities, because there it gets too cold for a homeless drunk. In those places you could freeze to death.

In the big cities you could stay in restaurants or the bus station. You wouldn't want to waste money on a place to live because you need that money for booze. That's why I moved West, where it was warmer and I could sleep outside. I wouldn't stay in the missions because they'd make you come in at seven o'clock and leave at seven in the morning. As an alcoholic, I couldn't be sobering up that early in the evening. Sometimes I slept in restaurants or hotel lobbies, but usually in a parking lot. All you need in that wine world is a Tokay blanket. As long as you have a bottle of Tokay, you don't feel the cold. There're a lot of places that give out free clothes or meals so the homeless won't starve to death, but lots of days I was too sick to eat anything. When I'd go to jail, I couldn't eat or drink untill I'd gone through the D.T.s.

On skid row there were also places to take showers, and I always tried to shave and keep clean. I always thought one day I was going to impress somebody, and as long as I stayed cleaned up, they wouldn't think I was a drunk. Maybe they'd hire me for a good job or put me into the movies. It's ironic because after I won the Sundance case, Twentieth Century Fox twice tried to get me to sign a contract for my story and I turned them down because their scripts weren't true. They were too fictional, and I wanted to show the true ordeals of my journey. I didn't want to make alcoholism and drunks a big joke. I wanted to show the facts.

The worst part of the ordeal was being so damn sick in the mornings. If I stood up too fast, I'd start to black out. I'd have to sit down again until somebody brought me a drink. Then I'd get stronger, but it was the same way the next morning again, and it just got worse. I want young alcoholics to know that having a drink to get going may seem like it's alleviating the problem, but really it gets worse and worse and never gets better. Alcoholism is insidious. You fool yourself. Defense mechanisms cause you always to blame someone else and make you think you're doing the right thing. Everyone else is wrong.

In Jail and Fighting the System

In Los Angeles, I was arrested for public drunkenness about 300 times, and a couple hundred times around the country besides. I repeatedly asserted that I was "not guilty." The sentences in the 60s were 120 days, and anybody who got 30 days felt that they got off scott-free. If you pled not guilty and changed your plea to guilty, they'd turn you loose, but I wouldn't do that. I wanted a trial, and the court administrators wouldn't give me one, not a single trial in ten years. They denied me my constitutional right to a jury trial because they knew they were wrong and didn't want the public to know about it. The power mongers didn't want to let me be heard in court, because if I won—as I eventually did—it would outlaw the barbarous practice of locking up public inebriates.

Public defenders routinely sold me out. They'd threaten and say anything to get me to plead guilty. They tried to bribe me, saying that I'd only have to serve one day if I'd plead guilty, but I stuck to my principles. What's more, when they let you go, they'd turn around and arrest you again the same night. At the time there were only two or three facilities for rehabilitating alcoholics, but they wouldn't send me to a facility. I wanted to go to one of the programs because I heard that they could make you stop drinking and keep you out of jail. The lawyers told me that the only way I could get sent for rehabilitation would be if I pled guilty, which was repugnant to me. One time, when I was told by the P.D.s that if I pled guilty they would send me to a rehabilitation facility, I was afraid and didn't trust them; but since they kept promising me that they'd send me, I finally took the chance. I said, "Guilty," and the judge sentenced me to 100 days and one year probation. They had to drag me, protesting, out of the courtroom. I would never again plead guilty. The public defender never helped me, and the only reason I ever again used one was to witness the recording of my sentence. I didn't want to plead "not guilty" and have them write down "guilty." A few times I pled *no lo contendre,* which basically amounted to pleading guilty, because I was so sick I had to get out to have a drink.

A lot of times I'd be in jail for three or four months, not drinking, and I never received medical attention, which is why I got the D.T.s so many times. The position of the authorities was, "You're just a damn drunk, suffer." I saw guys die in jail; and, without even knowing who they were, their remains were cremated. The drunk tank would be stuffed with about 140 drunks, and a lot of alcoholics used different names. If they didn't recognize you or know your name, with all of the overcrowding, they'd give you a "kick out." Jail was a hell of an ordeal.

When I'd get out, I'd go get a drink, and pretty soon they'd come and arrest me again. I'd drink and hold out for as long as I could, hiding from the police, but they'd recognize me and whenever they saw me I got arrested.

For all those years I never got mail. I never voted. I was in jail for seven of the last ten years of my drinking career on "not guilty" pleas. I would not even stipulate probable cause, because to me that would have justified an illegal arrest by the police. I contended that alcoholism is a disease and to jail a physically ill, chronic alcoholic, especially an indigent one, because he has no home, violates the United States Constitution's Eighth Amendment ban on cruel and unusual punishment. To jail a sick person is a barbarous practice, like locking someone up for diabetes. I've always contended that if homeless, public inebriates, who are on the lowest rung of society's totem pole, can be locked up, then they can lock up any other class as well.

In the meantime I was writing petitions. I wrote eighty petitions in ten years. When I was in jail, I went to the library and read everything I could, especially on law. I learned how to do legal work, and used a dictionary to learn to spell and correctly pronounce legal words. I had to write my petitions with a pencil on yellow paper, if I was fortunate enough to get it. A legal pad of paper would be my prized possession. All I did in jail was write and read. I wouldn't play dominos or sports. I wouldn't watch television because I wanted to be productive in my struggle. I wrote letters for other inmates who were illiterate, and in exchange they'd buy me stamps and legal tablets. I had to copy everything by hand. There were no copier machines; in fact, I didn't even know that xerox machines existed.

The whole system was in on a conspiracy to continue unconstitutionally and immorally arresting and jailing sick alcoholics. The judges would stamp my petitions "Denied" without even considering them. They were upholding an inhumane practice while misusing millions of dollars of taxpayers' money for transporting the drunks, keeping them in jail, and processing them through the courts. In 1975, the year the Sundance case was filed, there were 50,595 arrests for public drunkenness in Los Angeles, opposed to 1,113 in 1984 after the effects of the Sundance case were substantially felt. Of course, in 1975, it was the same 2,500 or so exploited people getting arrested over and over. To the public, the figures seemed like the police were doing a wonderful job locking up real criminals and keeping society safe.

The system used us as slave labor, making us work for free. If someone had a skill they'd be picked up again as soon as they got out of jail. Cooks and plumbers were in especially bad shape. I've seen guys given a few bucks when they were released, with the authorities knowing they were alcoholics and that they'd immediately go get a drink. Then the L.A.P.D. would trail these guys and pick them up again as soon as they'd had a few drinks. One guy who was a cabinet maker, a master craftsman, used to get sentences of 180 days. They'd put him to work making cabinets, then turn around and sell his handiwork without giving him a penny. When I asked him why he went along with it, he was dumbfounded. He didn't realize that he could say "No."

The court process was a sham. They'd run 350 of us through there in a few hours. In 1974, one courtroom handled 29,780 cases for public drunkenness, and in that year not a single case went to trial. In that year, I was in jail 277 days, 125 of which were spent supposedly awaiting trial on "not guilty" pleas. Each time my case would come up for trial, I would be released for insufficient evidence. There was no reason for them to try my case because I had already served longer than my sentence would be. My case went unheard. Entire arraignments lasted only about three minutes. A lot of those guys didn't even realize that they didn't have to plead guilty. I'd tell them, "Just plead not guilty," but they wouldn't. We could have had 300 jury trials per day, which would have broken the back of the system, but the other drunks would not stand with me and plead not guilty. The system is smart because they'd let guys out in three or five days if they'd plead guilty to public drunkenness. I wouldn't, so they kept me for thirty.

Almost all of my Los Angeles arrests were for violating Penal Code section 647(f), which makes it a misdemeanor to be drunk in a public place. The other times were for begging. Once, a cop asked me what I was doing, and I told him I was trying to find a dime to make a phone call. He said I asked him for a dime and wrote me up for begging. I pled not guilty and stayed in jail for thirty days before they let me out without a trial. The other time I was on my way to unload a semi-trailer. I was pretty sick, but I wanted the money. Some guy called out to me. He was wearing dirty clothes and had a flat top: he looked like a regular wino. He asked me where I was going, and I explained about the job. He tried to convince me to have a drink with him, but I told him I wasn't interested in having a drink, I just wanted to make that money. He said, "A drink won't hurt you, let's chip in." I said I had a quarter and just wanted to get a nickel more so I could ride the bus to where the trailer was going to be unloaded. I said, "I'm getting late now, but if you give me a nickel, I can still get there on time." He then told me that he was an undercover policeman and arrested me for begging. I was in jail on that one for another thirty days.

Besides the legal system itself, the liquor industry must take a huge share of the blame. The liquor lobby has a lot of clout with the politician. Think of the millions of dollars spent on beer and wine advertising. That represents a small fraction of the investment that these people have in keeping alcohol flowing. They're especially intent upon deceiving young kids into believing that they'll be great sports heroes, attractive like the models, or romantic and adventurous. When young people start drinking, they have no idea of the possible horrors; but, the more they drink, the more it alters their perceptions about reality and themselves.

In 1971, I sent one of my petitions for a *writ of habeus corpus* to Judge Warren J. Ferguson of the U.S. District Court. I didn't know him, but the guys in jail said he was honorable. Legally, you must exhaust your remedies to the state courts first, but they weren't reading my writs. I decided to send this particular petition along anyway. It was just mediocre, not even one of my better petitions, but the lawyers and judge thought it was outstanding. I knew that Judge Ferguson would deny it, though, because I by-passed channels. He did dismiss it, but he added the words, "This court reluctantly dismisses . . ." which indicated to me that he thought I was right. Hurriedly, I started in again, but the authorities kept me in and out of jail and wanted to send me to a mental institution where they could have kept me indefinitely. Plus, as they kept arresting me, I'd have my papers taken from me. I had no home and nowhere safe to leave them, so they would be lost. Between 1972 and 1975, I spent an average of 226 days in jail per year.

In April of 1975, I sent out my eightieth petition, and again cut across normal channels by sending it to Judge Ferguson, who again denied the petition, as was required by jurisprudence. However, he sent a copy of it to the Center for Law in the Public Interest. No lawyers wanted to take on a skid row issue with a bunch of derelicts. In fact, even the American Civil Liberties Union and Indian lawyers refused to have anything to do with my case. Of course, after I won at the Superior Court level, everyone wanted to represent me. Anyway, five or six lawyers at the Center passed my letter along without wanting to have anything to do with it. Finally, Timothy B. McFlynn, who had only been there for six weeks, got interested.

He visited me in jail, and I had all of my papers there with me. In all those years, I had never had a visitor. He had long hair and a beard, and I was afraid he was some kind of hippie or a plant from the police department. I was leery about showing him my papers because I feared he might tear them up. So, from memory, I recited about 150 different precedents, citations, pages, and cases. He brought a stenographer with him, who wrote down everything. McFlynn had no idea that this kind of exploitation existed, though he should have because he had been a prosecuting attorney. We spent about three and a half hours together, and he decided to check out what I had told him. Eventually, after he realized that everything I had told him was true, he took the case. A complaint was finally filed against the Los Angeles Police Department, et al., in July of 1975.

Recovery and Changing the System

This is where my recovery began. In taking my case, McFlynn wanted to get me out of jail and into a rehabilitation program. I had to be sober for the trial. It was the first time in thirty years I ever got bailed out. I was released on a Friday, but couldn't get into the program until Monday. A social worker had arranged for a place I could stay that weekend, but I wanted to walk around a little. I started talking to a couple of friends, and pretty soon a paddy wagon came with police hanging on it like Keystone Cops. They arrested all of us as drunks, and I hadn't even had a drink yet. Neither had the other two. One of them was just coming from jail and had money. He wanted to go get a drink and I told him that I was staying off of it to go to the program. They charged the other two guys with drunkenness but arrested me for begging; so I couldn't get kicked-out on Sunday and go into the program. The social worker bailed me out again, and the same thing happened one more time before I finally got to the rehabilitation center.

Warm Springs was a Los Angeles County facility in the mountains and it really had a wonderful program. I was there for 100 days and, although I sincerely wanted to quit, I still snuck drinks. The guy who bunked next to me had smuggled in vodka, and I figured if he could handle it, so could I. When I was caught drunker than hell, they threw me out of the program and dumped me at the bus station in downtown Los Angeles. That night I got thrown into jail again. I was thrown into jail twelve more times before I got into another rehabilitation facility.

My social worker looked for programs and got me into Harbor Light, right in the heart of skid row. I thought back to some of the old drunks at Warm Springs who were making it. In Harbor Light, I knew I could walk out at any time and get a drink. There was a liquor store right across the street, and I had some money. I thought I would never be able to make it. They said they wanted me to stay sober for three days, which seemed impossible, but I toughed it out and stayed with the program. All the others in there were alcoholics. Some of them were old drinking buddies of mine. They were all cleanly dressed and looked happy and seemed like big shots. That's what I wanted to be like instead of always hustling a drink.

Nobody can motivate you to go into a program. It's the program that motivates you. I went in with a lot of hostility. I thought I knew everything because booze does that to you. You get false courage and if things don't go your way, there's always the bottle. The program taught me that it didn't have to be that way. They helped me see the reasons why I drank, and helped me to learn that I didn't have to drink. Reluctantly, I went along with it and thought I'd stay a while. The longer I stayed, the more I learned. Listening to those other guys talk, I saw that I wasn't the only one who got so damn sick, and that the police picked on all of the drunks, not just me. Believe me, they did pick on me, especially because of my mission and goal of bringing my case to trial.

A month went by, and I kept hearing them talk about what booze does to you and the problems that it causes. They were slowly convincing me that I wouldn't have to go through all of that pain again if I could stay sober. If you can keep the booze out of your system, and want to stay sober, then you have a chance. You barely get sober in thirty days, but after ninety days I started to feel pretty good. Sobriety is not recovery; there is still a long way to go. I was sober for long periods of time in jail, but I still had the same habits I'd lived with all of my life. As an alcoholic, I constantly conned people, I hustled, schemed, and ripped others off. If you're just sober, then you're a sober thief or sober con-artist. I had a hard time understanding that to be recovered, those traits had to go. I thought that once I was sober, I'd be cured, but an alcoholic is never really cured.

I began using other coping skills instead of using drinking. Whenever I got angry as an alcoholic, I reached for a drink as a way to escape. In recovery, I wouldn't do that. Instead, I got angry at the system and thought of all the wrongs they had done to me. I was in court all of this time with the Sundance case and when I was under pressure, I would imagine myself changing the system. I replaced alcohol with my political, judicial mission.

After a year, my head started clearing up and the bad habits began to fade. For two years I stayed on antabuse, which makes you very sick if you drink alcohol. I wanted to find a way not to have to drink anymore, so I could eventually walk free without any crutch—not A.A., church, or antabuse. I've been able to do it, but first I had to get off of alcohol. The cravings to drink continued for about two years. My body screaming for a drink was the toughest part. It took at least ten years to really walk free, especially working around skid row.

I stayed in the program for two years and was hired to be night supervisor. I ran the facility, was responsible for security, and essentially ran the place. I had a place to stay and food to eat. I went to weekly meetings. At the start I went to Alcoholics Anonymous meetings, but I didn't like the anonymity. I wanted to shout to the world that I was an alcoholic and that the liquor industry had hooked me with their fallacious advertising and the implied promises that booze would make me successful. It was mandatory in the program to go to three A.A. meetings each week, and I went to occasional lectures as well. I also attended bureaucratic political meetings on alcoholism, which is how I came into contact with the Indian Alcoholism Commission of California, of which I am now the Executive Director.

Alcoholism is destroying the whole Indian race. Even those who don't drink are affected by it. That's why I'm trying to alleviate the problem before it's too late. I'm trying to promote sobriety among American Indian nations of this country. That's the only way we're going to survive and ever regain our rightful place in this country. Sobriety is the secret of success for the Indian people as well as the rest of society.

On December 5, 1977, in Los Angeles Superior Court, Judge Harry L. Hupp presented an 87 page memorandum opinion in my favor, and to the great benefit of skid row alcoholics. I won! A national precedent was established, and within ten years 35 states had decriminalized public drunkenness. Ironically, California was not one of them. Among the results of the Sundance case, the city and county of Los Angeles were given a mandate to upgrade jail facilities, police who arrested individuals for public drunkenness had to take them to an alcoholism facility, and if no facility was available, they were to be carefully watched through detoxification and given proper nutritional guidance. Arrests for public drunkenness were dramatically cut to 2% within five years. My United States Supreme Court case asks that the jailing of alcoholics be declared unconstitutional. I'm now waiting for them to decide whether to hear the case.

I don't regret the past, the wasted years. Without those experiences, I would probably have settled down somewhere, raised a family, and lived an unspectacular life. I'm tremendously proud of my accomplishments. My case has saved the Los Angeles taxpayers many millions of dollars by stopping the police from locking up alcoholics. I've changed the way the police focus on drunks, which used to waste time and money. Now they can concentrate on real criminals and do their duty to serve and protect. Now there're many facilities on skid row for alcoholics and the homeless. Regardless of the results of my efforts in the U.S. Supreme Court, I will never give up my assault on the inadequacies of society.

I believe that alcoholism is never cured. If I had a drink now, I'd be right back down there. Maybe I would hold out for some time, but then I'd have another one because that stuff makes you feel good. If I had kept on drinking, I would have died drunk, and my whole life would have been without meaning.

ANOREXIA NERVOSA

About the Author

Avis Rumney might skip breakfast, eat a salad or sandwich for lunch (but only if she had exercised heavily beforehand) and then would skip dinner. This was her typical eating pattern for 17 years of anorexia nervosa. Her obsession with thinness made her feel that even at 68 pounds she could still be thinner.

Most of the time she was too depressed to eat; and, antidepressants, therapy, and marriage did not fill her emptiness or provide her with a sense of direction. Food was a reward, and she rarely felt deserving. She viewed her amenorrhea as a convenient form of birth control and her ability to go without food as a way to save money. She refused to acknowledge her eating disorder as a problem, and when she eventually entered treatment for her depression, she was offended to be diagnosed an anorexic.

Avis Rumney has been at a normal weight for more than nine years. She now enjoys her work, relationships, meals, and time alone. Her perfectionism has been replaced by a quest for personal fulfillment and an ongoing process of self-discovery. She is a Marriage, Family and Child Counselor specializing in eating disorders and is the author of a book on anorexia nervosa.

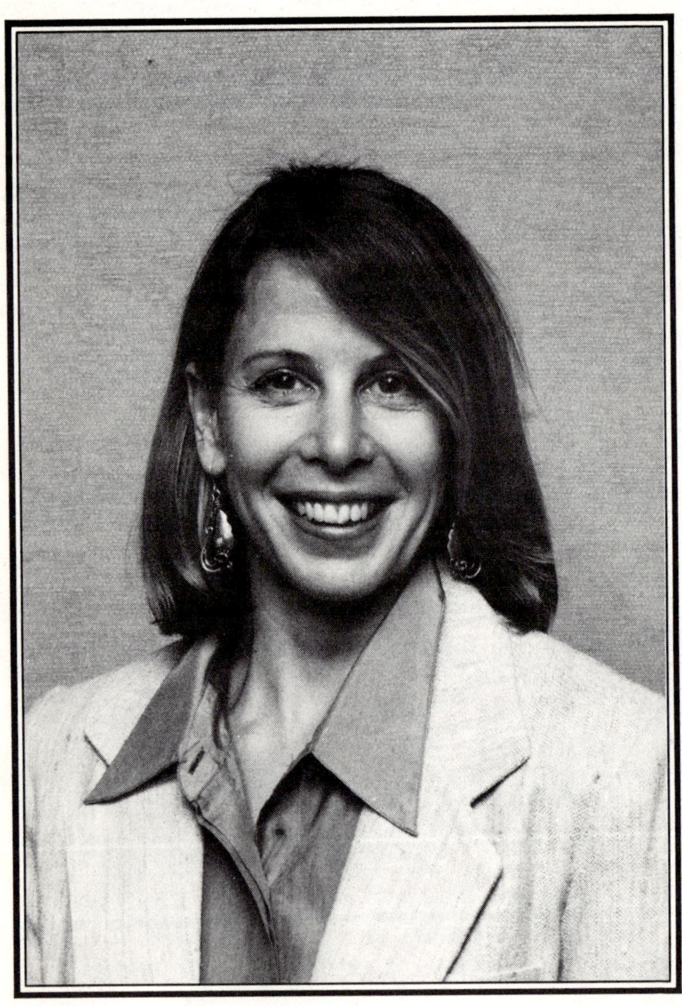

Avis Rumney

Soul Starvation

by

Avis Rumney

***

Breakfast

It's a warm, sunny August morning in San Rafael, the kind of day I like to spend at home doing things I enjoy. Sitting on the back deck, bathed in Summer sunlight, sipping herb tea, I relax to the sounds of birds chirping in the bushes and neighbors chatting over Saturday chores. My eyes wander admiringly over my garden of colorful potted plants, geraniums, impatiens and brachycome in shades of lavender and pink. Later I'll sweep the deck and cut some flowers to put in a vase. When I'm in a hurry in the mornings, I may only grab a muffin and a piece of cheese, gaze for a moment out the kitchen window at my flowers, and rush off to work or appointments. But, today I can take my time. This morning I fixed one of my favorite breakfasts of scrambled eggs with mushrooms, onions, and cheese; buttered, whole wheat toast; and bacon, and ate breakfast at a leisurely pace with my boyfriend Rick.

When I first came to the Bay Area nine years ago, I was a vegetarian and would not have eaten the bacon. Actually, I would not have eaten anything. I weighed 68 pounds; and, for the 17 years I was anorexic, breakfast was rarely a part of my vocabulary. I hardly ever ate in the mornings, and I only allowed myself food after I ran for thirty or forty minutes or swam a half mile. Eating was a reward for exhausting myself with physical exercise, or for enduring the pain of hunger for at least a day. Now, food is something I enjoy. I like many different foods, and I enjoy their different tastes and textures. Food gives me energy and nourishment. I don't deprive myself of food anymore. I get hungry at intervals throughout the day and I eat when I'm hungry.

I appreciate the sun and my garden and look forward to the rest of my day. When I was anorexic, not only did I deny myself food, but I could not feel relaxed or peaceful. I've changed so much since I came to the Bay Area for treatment. Most obvious is my appearance. My weight has stabilized at around 102 to 105 pounds since I was in therapy and contracted with my therapists to eat more. Now, that weight feels comfortable on my 5'2" frame. However, the more significant changes are less outwardly apparent. I accept myself—as a person, as a woman—in a way that I could not even imagine ten years ago. I like my work as a Marriage, Family and Child Counselor, specializing in treating people with eating disorders; and, I enjoy myself without worrying so much about who I am or what I should be doing.

Tonight, some good friends are coming over for a barbecue. Actually, "barbecue" doesn't really do justice to the meal we've planned. Rick and I will smoke an organic turkey over mesquite in our Weber, and I'll create a delicious stuffing with bread crumbs, sauteed mushrooms and onions, walnuts, raisins and wild rice. We will also serve hors d'oeuvres of herb and salsa and cheese dips with tortilla chips, mashed potatoes with gravy, corn on the cob, salad, and carrot cake with cream cheese frosting. I'll eat some of everything and savor every bite! Dinner will be like a Thanksgiving feast in August.

I have a lot for which to be thankful, but most of all, I think my recovery has given me the ability to have fun, especially with other people. Ten years ago, I did not know the meaning of "close friends." I was much too concerned about what other people thought of me to trust that I could *like* anyone, or they me. And I was convinced as little as three years ago, that I would never be able to have a satisfactory relationship with a man, much less to be able to *love* someone and believe he loved me. I thought in a relationship I was doomed to be the self-effacing martyr I thought my mother was with my father, and to be unhappy in love, as in life.

Growing Up

My childhood was not particularly pleasant. I don't think I was always depressed as a child, but I just wasn't happy. I was forever wondering who I was and what I was supposed to be doing, which were the same questions that haunted me for most of my life. I never felt secure from moment to moment. I had the sense that other kids somehow knew how to have fun, but I didn't. I could play with my dolls or ride my bike, but that never gave me the kind of enjoyment I saw other kids having.

Actually, I don't think my family was ever really into fun. We always had enough of everything, like food and clothing, though we didn't get a television until I was a twelve, and then there were strict rules about how much TV we kids could watch each day. We lived in a nice house, but emotionally it seemed fairly bleak. My father worked diligently as a university professor, and after classes, he would return home to grade papers and prepare for the next day. My mother had been a librarian, and went back to work part-time when I was about ten, but during my younger years she was primarily a housewife and mother. I sensed that both my parents spent all of their time working. My father was pretty much the silent ruler of the house—not that he was authoritarian—but my mother tried to please him. When I asked why we had dinner at 6:00 every night, she replied, "Because that's what your father likes."

At dinner, my father was quiet and reserved and didn't converse much with the rest of us. He was also an alcoholic. His drinking problem was not obvious, and probably didn't become severe until I was twelve or thirteen. My mother was very controlling around meals, and she would hop up and down taking care of everyone and everything. She dished the food out in the kitchen, and we'd sit in the dining room. If anyone wanted anything, she'd jump up from the table and get it. In the evenings, my mother would clean up the kitchen. She wouldn't let me help because, "My mother never let me help when I was your age," and then later, she would plop in a chair, exhausted, to read for a little while. My father would continue his paperwork, or sometimes read the evening newspaper. I guess my brothers went to their rooms and me to mine, to do homework or read. I don't remember ever *talking about* what we read with each other. Occasionally, on the weekends, we went for drives in the country, but that was boring. Looking back, I don't remember being excited by much of anything in childhood.

My twin brother, Adrian, and I were constant companions in early childhood, playing and fighting with each other. As we grew older, Adrian preferred to spend time by himself. I had few friends and so was alone a lot, too. By high school, we had outgrown the fighting, but we didn't get along very well. Adrian was smarter than I was, and with the minimum amount of effort he got better grades than I did. If I had a problem with my homework, I'd ask him for help, and usually get it, but half the time I didn't really understand his explanations, and I felt like a real dummy having to ask him in the first place. Sometimes I wondered if I'd been brought home as a baby to the wrong house; both my brothers and my parents were so smart, and I always felt out of their league. I'm sure that my parents admired Adrian's brilliance. He could play chess when he was six and could solve puzzles in seconds. He didn't do the minimal chores around the house that he was supposed to do, and even though I was helpful, I never found that it made much difference. The "thank you, dear" 's always left me with a momentary glow, and then a gnawing, persistent emptiness.

I looked up to my older brother, George. He was two years older, and I admired him because he was both smart *and* sociable. Also, he seemed warmer than other members of my family. I felt a security and perhaps an availability from him that I didn't get from my father. George had lots of friends, and I envied the way he seemed able to get a kick out of life. Nobody else in the family seemed to have a handle on that!

The person I remember with the most fondness from my childhood is my maternal grandmother. We'd visit my grand-parents in New Jersey for vacations, and I would spend a lot of time around her then. She made me feel invaluable, and even when I did small things, like setting the table, she'd say, "I don't know how I ever got along without you." She cared about me and always to gave me the kind of attention that I lacked at home. I realize now, that as a grandparent and not a parent, she didn't have to deal with a lot of the disciplinary and day-to-day stuff that my parents did. Although I believed I was not good, smart, or pretty enough, to my grandmother, I was just right.

When I was thirteen, my grandmother became ill and died. I didn't know how to deal with her death. Losing her upset me, but it also triggered those same questions of wondering what I should be feeling and doing. My mother went back East for the funeral, and she asked me to help out around the house while she was gone, so I did what I thought she meant. I fixed everyone's breakfast and packed lunches for my brothers; and, after school, I cleaned and cooked, but I felt entirely helpless. I never knew if I was doing these things correctly or even what I was supposed to be doing. Whatever feelings I had about my mother being gone and my grandmother's dying were suppressed because I was a little robot trying to take care of everything. Although my father and brothers appreciated my efforts, they were used to having it all done for them anyway. I was just a substitute robot to them! No matter how much I did, I knew that it wasn't enough. After my mother returned, she resumed her role as the homemaker. For all my efforts, nothing seemed to matter and I was left with more uncertainty and emptiness. At that point, I knew I did not want the kind of life my mother had.

Around that time, another critical incident occurred. To any other kid, it might have been just a small matter, but it provoked me to stop eating. Ours was a food-centered household, and I used to come home from school for lunch, and after school to milk and cookies set out for me by my mother. I suppose that my sense of security was supposed to come from the food instead of from her because she would leave the table to get on with her housework. One particular day while my mother was away on errands at lunch-time, I helped myself to extra servings of left-over sweets. When she got home, I proudly exclaimed, "I just had three desserts!" Instead of sharing my pleasure, she remarked critically with a furrowed brow and a frown on her face, "You're going to be fat!" Bruised and afraid to say anything out loud in reply, I thought, "I'll show you! I'm not going to gain weight!" After that incident, I harbored a tremendous resentment towards her and a burning desire to prove her wrong.

I was already conscious of my weight. I was a slow developer and, in adolescence, was on the chubby side. My body shape most closely resembled a barrel and I was padded with baby fat in all the wrong places. When I went to high school, chronologically younger than many of my classmates, and still younger developmentally , I saw that many of the girls in the locker room had figures already. I reasoned that the only way to have a thin waist like theirs was by dieting—if my plump middle got smaller, and the top and the bottom got added to, or just stayed the same, then I'd look more like the other girls did. Also, I thought that boys were noticing me. Their attention made me feel awkward and terribly embarrassed. I imagined that if I could lose weight from all the bad places and put it on in all the right ones, then maybe I would look like I fit in better, and I wouldn't feel so out of place.

Shedding Pounds

I began to consciously diet, and devised ways to eat less without being noticed. I don't really know what would have happened if I said I *wanted* to eat less and be thinner, but I did not want to give the control back to my mother. I was determined to lose weight on my own. Also my mother was always dieting but she never seemed to succeed. I wanted my diet to *work!* I started to skip breakfast, but I made it appear as though I had already eaten. I arose before the rest of the family, put crumbs on a plate, poured milk in a glass and then back in the milk carton, and then left my dirty plate and glass in the sink. My father played a similar game. He had an early morning drink from a liquor bottle he kept in a tool cabinet in the pantry. We had an unspoken pact, "If you don't tell on me, I won't tell on you." I'm not sure if he knew what I was doing, but he didn't ask. Nor did I ask him about his drinking, or at least, not any more. On a vacation the summer before, Adrian and I found a half empty bottle of Scotch hidden under the driver's seat of the family car, and we asked my mother about it. She replied, "Well, just put it back. Your father gets thirsty sometimes." Then the matter was dropped. The meaning was clear enough to me, "Don't ask." Although I did not understand what was happening at the time, because my father was an alcoholic he was preoccupied with hiding his alcohol dependency, just as I, an anorexic, was hiding my food dependency.

I also threw away most of my school lunches, eating only a piece of fruit or a couple of carrot sticks. The milk and cookies were no longer left by my mother, who was working afternoons, so I stopped having snacks when I got home. I read that eating fruit could help with weight loss, so before dinner I usually smuggled a couple of oranges or a grapefruit upstairs to eat in my bedroom. That helped to fill me up and to prevent hunger from getting the best of me at dinner. Then I went downstairs to set the table and serve milk for my brothers and me. I poured some milk out of a glass in the kitchen and then claimed that I had drunk mine already. At dinner, I discreetly shoveled most of my meal into my napkin. Then I surreptitiously emptied my napkin into the trash and cleaned it off as best I could. We used cloth napkins, and mine always became particularly soggy. My plan worked, and I lost weight steadily.

My parents became concerned about my unexplained weight loss and took me to the family doctor, who did blood tests and gave me a complete physical. He said that if I didn't gain weight, I'd have go into the hospital. That scared me into eating enough to get everyone off my back.

I no longer appeared to have anorexia nervosa. Yet, I still had no sense of me as a person, and no sense of future. By the age of twelve, Adrian already knew he was going to be a mathematician; but, even when I finished high school, I didn't have the slightest idea what I wanted and I envied him for having it all figured out. I pretty much assumed that, like my mother, I'd get married and have kids, which was not an appealing thought. I don't know how conscious at this time was either my fear of growing up and being just like her—looking like her, having a life like hers—or my determination to intervene with that process by controlling my body and not allowing myself to get fat.

When I went away to college at sixteen, I followed a family tradition. My brothers went to the same school as my father, and I went to Mt. Holyoke in Massachusetts, a private girls' college, which was my mother's alma mater. I suppose I chose Mt. Holyoke mostly because if it was right for my mother, then it should be right for me. I didn't really have any idea how to choose; I wasn't even sure there *was* a me other than who I thought my parents wanted me to be. The situation at college was horrible. I was desperately homesick and depressed. To make matters worse, my dormitory roommate was a bouncy, eighteen year old socialite. She had probably been dating since she was eight; and, although I dated a little in high school (and was even elected junior prom queen one year when I was one of three junior girls who had a *date* to the prom), I was clearly out of my league. She looked like she had stepped out of the pages of *Glamour Magazine*.. She had wavy, chestnut colored, shoulder length hair, a well-developed body, and a penchant for all-night partying. I was socially backward, and came from a conservative family in the Midwest. Being around her made me feel like a sixth grader. I petitioned for and was granted a single room my second semester, and it was then that I discovered what true isolation could be. I also began seeing the school psychiatrist because I became more and more depressed as the school year progressed. He was a friendly chap who immediately prescribed antidepressants for me, which I thought was a novel way to deal with what I perceived as my mixed up feelings. My brother, George was fairly nearby at Yale University, and long phone calls with him were my life line that year. He was the only person who really seemed to understand the torment I was going through, probably because he had experienced some dark moments his first year away at school. My calls to him were glimmers of light in an otherwise black existence.

With the combination of dorm food, depression and loneliness, I gained weight during my first semester at college. Now, not only did I feel miserable, I felt fat, too. By Spring, I began again to consciously limit how much food I ate. I avoided dorm meals whenever possible, skipping breakfast altogether and opting for a mid-afternoon ice cream cone from a sundae shop opposite the campus instead of lunch and dinner. This time my diet lasted for fourteen years.

After I graduated, my family had moved to Houston, Texas and summer vacation after my freshman year was wretched. I only knew three other girls my age in Houston, and they were all so "different" from me that it was like college all over again; I didn't fit in. One was rich, one was super religious, and one was socially light years ahead of me. For part of the summer, I worked at an excruciatingly boring clerical job copying zip codes for hours at a stretch. I thought I was going out of my mind, and wondered how any adult could tolerate working for a living.

The scene at home was as depressing as it had ever been. I think my father was nearing a crisis with his alcoholism and I found out that when I was in school that winter, he was on the verge of a nervous breakdown. I think my mother missed her old friends, and was upset about my father, because she seemed really unhappy, too. George had moved to New York City to work after graduation from college and didn't come home at all. Adrian was keeping pretty much to himself. I had hated college and now I hated being home. To add to my misery, I also had my wisdom teeth extracted during that summer. I'd seen George recover from having two wisdom teeth pulled out at a time. I didn't want to go through that agony twice, so I had all four removed at once. I knew recovery wasn't going to be comfortable, but I hadn't anticipated complications. However, one of the upper incisions got infected and instead of getting back to eating in three days, I lived on soup and milk shakes for over a week. My weight had been fairly normal for my size when vacation started, probably around 100 pounds, but I quickly lost several more. There was not much that I liked about my life then *except* being lighter, and I decided not to regain the weight.

School in the fall was just as bad as it had been before, only now George was far away in New York City and busy with his new job. I felt even more lost. I had dated one of his friends who also moved to New York, so at the end of the first semester, I quit school and moved to the big city. My parents wanted me to come home to Houston, but with the problems my father was having, and memories of how miserable I had been there the previous summer, I would not even consider going home. Initially, I lived in a Village loft George shared with his artist roommate, but when George was drafted into the army, I had to move out. I was eighteen, and found low-paying clerical jobs from the first week I was there. I wanted to make it on my own and would not take money from my parents, but the jobs I found were barely enough to live on.

During most of that time, I didn't really have enough money to buy food. In part my poor finances were just an excuse for not eating. My parents, or the aunt and uncle I saw occasionally in New York, would have given me money for food, had I been willing to ask them, but I was rebellious and determined to survive without anyone's help. I allowed myself one meal per day, a sandwich from the deli near where I worked. Having not eaten since lunch the previous day, at noon I would race to the deli around the corner, order an egg salad and bacon sandwich, and rush back to the office cafeteria to devour my meal for the day. I think the man behind the counter at the deli felt sorry for me, because some days there would be extra pickles, or more bacon than usual, or the sandwich would be extra stuffed. That's all I ate, and I maintained this routine for months. Food was my reward, and I rarely permitted myself more, even when I was tremendously hungry.

Ironically, my job as junior secretary to the executive offices of Maidenform, Inc. entitled me to a discount on all the brassieres and girdles I wanted to buy. But at 80 pounds with no breasts or hips to speak of, these undergarments were superfluous. At the time I thought it was a shame to have this buying opportunity wasted on me—if only I had found a job at Bloomingdale's or Saks Fifth Avenue where a store discount would have been useful!

I hated the clerical jobs I was able to get as a college drop out, and knew I had to finish school to get better employment. Even though I still had no idea what I wanted to do with my life, I enrolled at NYU hoping that I miraculously would find some direction.

While at NYU, I met Michael, who seemed interesting , and more important, was interested in me. He was 13 years my senior, English, intellectual, and charming. Within a year Michael and I got married. My parents came to New York and hosted a small wedding, but they did not particularly care for Michael. On my wedding day I weighed only 75 pounds and was clearly anorexic.

Only one person seemed able to talk to me about my weight (or perhaps this was the only person I was willing to listen to): my brother, George. He came to meet Michael two months before the wedding, and told me that he was concerned about me. He asked how I would be able to manage my life being so thin. He also did not like Michael. His concerns filled me with doubts about myself and my decision to marry Michael, and I was haunted by feelings of guilt. George had always been the one to stand by me, and if *he* thought I was wrong, maybe there *was* something I was missing.

George did not come to my wedding. He said he didn't want to be around all the relatives, but I wondered if the real reason was because he disapproved of the match. Three weeks later, George committed suicide. I was plunged into despair and guilt. When George was discharged from the Army, he said he was planning to go to graduate school, but was been depressed for well over a year and suffered from the same kind of indecision that plagued me. He really did not know what he wanted to do with his life. I don't know for sure why he killed himself, but I think it had to do with his belief that he could not live up to my parents' expectations. Much later I heard a rumor that he had been a guinea pig for government drug testing while in the Army, but that was never substantiated. There have been many times in the years since that I have thought about taking my own life; but, George's death devastated my parents so much that I could never justify putting them through such grief again. Besides, I saw that his suicide accomplished nothing; and, although I often did not think life was worth living, I always hoped to find a greater purpose.

Searching for Myself

Married, depressed, and anorexic, I no longer avoided food for economic reasons. Now it was purely psychological. I didn't know any more about playing the role of a wife than I did about living any other part of my life. Michael commuted to a full time job and I went to classes during the day. I'd been given several cookbooks as wedding presents as well as lovely ceramic pots and pans, and I, who had never progressed much beyond boiling eggs at home, and that under the aegis of Girl Scouts, developed an interest in gourmet cooking. Michael returned home each evening to an elaborate dinner. I'd taste the food, but not eat it. I primarily lived on black coffee and cigarettes.

There was a certain degree of warmth in our marriage. Michael obviously cared about me and appreciated my intelligence. We were comfortable together and had an enjoyable sexual relationship. I liked the closeness in sex, but didn't really know what constituted sexual pleasure. The fact that I was not menstruating did not bother me, because I knew I couldn't handle having kids. I don't think I knew then that amenorrhea was a symptom of anorexia, and even if I had, I'm sure I would have denied any connection to my own circumstances. Michael became increasingly concerned about me. Anyone—except me—could see that I was too thin. In addition, I was only sleeping a couple of hours each night. Michael asked a friend to recommend a psychiatrist for me, and I had sessions with him once or twice every week and took the antidepressants he prescribed for me. This scenario continued for years: I saw a psychiatrist, was depressed and underweight. The depression did not change and neither did my weight. I stabilized at around 80 pounds, and rarely experienced hunger any longer.

During the first semester of my senior year at NYU, I was voted to Phi Beta Kappa for academic excellence. When it came time to get the award, I thought they had made some kind of mistake. I believed I did not deserve to be honored. I had struggled to study, but I knew I wasn't smart like George or Adrian. I had a low opinion of myself and had difficulty accepting praise. I felt unworthy at school, just as I did in the rest of my life, and I craved attention and reassurance from my professors. I'd latch onto teachers, hoping that one of them would give me the clue in my search for life's meaning. I changed my major three times depending on which professor gave me the most extra advice or recognition. Finally, I stuck with anthropology, because I had to take the fewest classes in that field to finish with a degree in that major. Even with the antidepressants, my last year of college was painfully difficult. Pressured by the anxiety of finishing my course work and terrified about what I was going to do after graduation (a B.A. in anthropology wasn't a great asset in the current job market), I remained depressed. I didn't know how to cope any other way.

As it turned out, my first three years after college were happier than I had expected. With the help of a cousin, I found a job as a scientific assistant in the Ichthyology Department of the American Museum of Natural History in New York. My boss appreciated my perfectionism and attention to detail. I liked him and was pleased that he thought I was doing a good job; although in my mind, my work was never quite "good enough." However, as a scientific assistant, I could not be promoted because a position as Curator required a Ph.D. Getting an advanced degree seemed like a logical next step. In the back of my mind was also the thought that I'd rather be doing something with more relevance to human beings than working with preserved fish. Perhaps I would become a teacher; after all, Adrian and my father were both college professors, so I knew that that was one way to make it in the world. Although I had more sense of direction in my life upon entering graduate school than before, in many ways school seemed a refuge, another place where I didn't have to decide yet what I wanted to be when—or if—I grew up.

I finished my Ph.D. course work, and received an M.A. in Biology along the way. However, the prospect of spending two years in a laboratory doing thesis research work did not appeal to me. I still didn't feel I was doing the "right thing." Something was missing, inside, and I was becoming severely depressed again. Michael did not know what he wanted to do with his life either. We decided to get out of New York and move to Provincetown, Massachusetts, but we were no longer getting along well together. Both of us were unhappy with our own lives, and neither of us could make it better for the other. He began seeing another woman, and we soon split up.

Whenever I had major upsets in my life—my grandmother's death, going away to college, dropping out of school, George's suicide, the breakup of my marriage—I had a sense of being lost, helpless, hopeless, not knowing what to do, and not knowing in what direction to turn. Each time, I stopped eating. And although losing weight was never my original motive, each time I stopped eating, I experienced secondary benefits. I *liked* the sensation of hunger, which enabled me to feel something in the face of bleak, grey, unfeeling depression. I *liked* the control, the knowledge that not eating was something I could *do*, and that this was an emptiness I was in charge of. I even liked being the recipient of other people's concern and attention.

To some extent, I was culturally influenced to be thin. Living in New York made me aware of fashion, and I admired nice clothes, which usually, it seems, were worn by thin women. I looked at popular women's magazines occasionally, and I would stare longingly in windows of Fifth Avenue department stores at emaciated mannequins wearing clothes too expensive to buy. I seldom watched television but I was envious of women in magazine pictures or in real life who always *appeared* to have their lives together. I lost weight mostly because not eating was something I knew how to do—a means of coping when I didn't know any other way. But also, I think I hoped that if somehow I could *look* more like other people who appeared to be thin and successful, maybe I would discover a clue to how to *be* successful myself.

Hitting Bottom

After separating from Michael, I moved into a place by myself at the opposite end of Provincetown from him. I was lonely, discouraged, and once again without a sense of future. I sold T-shirts that I'd hand-painted, and did some odd sewing jobs to make a little money, but mostly, I was depressed. Each afternoon, I swam for an hour in the chilling waters off Cape Cod, Icame home, took a long, hot shower to bring color back to my blue fingers and toes, and then ate a small but elaborate bowl of salad. That was my only meal of the day, and it was my reward for swimming. This was my daily ritual, and my weight dropped to the low 70's. I was addicted to the high I got from exercise, to the sense of power I got from not allowing myself to eat, and to the thinness—though I never did think I was thin enough.

For a short while, I saw a therapist who tried to work with me about my weight. He told me that he would not see me if I did not gain weight. I wasn't ready to handle this. As an excuse, I feigned illness, saying that I had the flu. He would have had a real control struggle with me if I had continued to work with him, but he moved away. Before he left, he recommended a treatment center in Oakland, California, and I stored away the information, not knowing if I would ever use it.

I drove across the country that fall, stored my belongings with Adrian, and went off to Hawaii to an herbal medicine retreat. Holistic medicine intrigued me—though as with many other pursuits previously, I wasn't sure it was for me, nor did I know how to make a paying job of it. The retreat did not work out, and I left with a low opinion of myself because I was unable to fit their methods into my life. Even though I was in a beautiful paradise, swimming every day in an ocean that was actually warm, basking in the sun, it was here that my life reached its lowest ebb.

I was travelling with a man who enjoyed life in the present and didn't worry about the future. Most of the time, he didn't know where his next meal was coming from or where he was staying that night. Ours was not a relationship with potential. I was drifting along without purpose with another drifter. My depression worsened again. In a desperate search to make some money and to feel functional, I took two jobs in Waikiki, one as a cocktail waitress at a restaurant, the other as a topless dancer at a bar. This was the most humiliating period of my life. It seemed so bizarre that the manager at the bar hired me. I weighed under 75 pounds and had nothing on top to show off, much less to bounce to the music. The money wasn't bad , and I didn't know where else to go, so I stayed for several months. Perhaps I wanted to punish myself, to see how bad off I could get. I didn't believe that I deserved any better. The hours were terrible. I was dancing from nine P.M. until three the next morning, and the bar was vile and smokey and always filled with rowdy Navy sailors. Although I have never been much of a drinker, I got a little drunk every night just to go on stage. That eased my embarrassment slightly, but I still felt like an awkward, underdeveloped, grotesque eleven year old. I admired the other dancers' bodies, but I was also convinced that if I ate, I would not look like them, I would look like my mother. And my mother's was not a body I liked much, nor did she.

Getting Help

I don't know what kept me going from one day to the next. There was nothing I viewed as positive about my life. Finally, with nowhere else to turn for help, I wrote to the people in Oakland that my therapist in Massachusetts recommended. I had trusted him and maybe that's why I kept the address. In my letter, I told them about my anxiety and depression, but did not mention my eating. I had no sense of being anorexic; my weight was not the issue to me. They accepted me into the program, and, at the age of thirty, I moved to the Bay Area with the fantasy of getting a good job and a nice apartment while in treatment on the side.

Cathexis Institute was oriented towards transactional-analysis. Group therapy and contractual agreements were the basis of treatment. Much of the work involved "reparenting", which meant the staff provided new, healthy parent messages to replace old information. Occasionally, staff members would make "contractual parent" agreements with program members to help them incorporate new ways of thinking and behaving. The therapist related emotionally to the client, and *vice versa,* as though the therapist were the client's parent.

I was offended from the very start. At the initial, diagnostic interview, the staff psychiatrist, David Kline, said to me, "With most of our patients, we have to ask what the problem is, but with you it's obvious." That stung me for a long time, because the problem was not obvious to me, and I certainly did not think it was my weight. How could he understand the emotional turmoil inside of my head by measuring my weight on a scale? I had no idea at the time that this man would play a significant role in my recovery or would later become my contractual father.

One of the first contracts I made with my treatment group was to gain one pound per week until I reached an amount determined in advance by the staff psychiatrist. I didn't agree that at 68 pounds I was underweight, and his proposed weight range for me of 100 to 108 pounds sounded like obesity incarnate. But I decided that I would go along with the program and gain the weight. They convinced me that they had an antidote to depression. However, I was determined that after treatment I would lose the weight again. By then, I wouldn't be depressed, I would have my life together, I could weigh 70 pounds if I wanted to!

I didn't look dehyrated although I was more than 30% under normal body weight. Many people at that stage of anorexia nervosa end up in hospitals, forcefed through tubes to their stomachs. If when I got to Cathexis, they had said, "You're severely underweight and the only way we'll work with you is if you agree to be hospitalized first," I probably would have run away. Maybe they had a backup plan for me if I didn't gain weight, but if they did, I never knew about it. Prior to going to Cathexis, I did not get close enough to anyone for them to care that much about me. I stayed away from my family, I had no close friends, and the man I traveled with in Hawaii did not have the capacity to see my pain. For me to have been hospitalized would have required that someone recognize that I was dangerously anorexic and confront me about it.

The first few months were frightening, because I didn't know who to trust. I was convinced that there was a conspiracy to make me fat—literally, every therapist on staff there was overweight, and not just by my anorexic standards! But I couldn't envision going back to the life I had had before. I had to suspend my distrust long enough to give this place a chance.

I ate three meals each day. I had never been much of a calorie counter while I was not eating. However, I was told I had to count calories—and worse, consume them—in order to gain weight. My psychiatrist helped me figure out how many calories I needed to eat each day. If I did not gain the prescribed pound each week, I had to eat more. I recorded everything I ate in a log. If I wasn't eating what I had contracted to eat, I was placed on food supervision. That meant it was my responsibility to ask a therapist or authorized program member to observe me weigh, measure, and eat every one of my meals for a week. I adapted to the new structure around eating, and only had to go on food supervision a couple of times.

I attributed much of my willingness to stay in the program and to continue gaining weight to my therapist, Tyanne Steckel. I had been immediately drawn to this woman when she interviewed me for the program. Much later in my treatment, she became my contractual mother. Tyanne was warm and nurturing, as well as strong and direct. She didn't hesitate to confront me when she thought it necessary. I needed both the softness and the firmness. She provided me with the encouragement I needed to stay in treatment. After I had been in Oakland for two weeks, she was coincidentally looking for a boarder to rent an extra room in her house. I originally wanted to have my own apartment, but the Institute required that I live in approved housing with other people in the program. Two weeks in a board and care facility had convinced me that other quarters were preferable. I moved in with Tyanne. Fortunately, my natural mother and father were able to help me by paying for my therapy and living expenses.

My purpose in living with Tyanne was not to get additional therapy from her, but that is what happened. She lived and breathed therapy, and that helped me tremendously. For one thing, Tyanne could not tolerate my being in her house and not eating. I'd sit down to dinner, and she would say, "Avis, you can't eat like that, eat like the rest of us!" And I would, partly because I trusted that she knew what was best for me, and partly because I had discovered that I actually liked some of the foods I had deprived myself of for so many years! I was scared of getting fat and gaining weight too fast, but Tyanne reminded me to use the structure I had learned about counting calories to determine how much to eat.

Tyanne was also a valuable role model for me. She had fun both exercising and relaxing. She enjoyed exercise because she liked how it felt. I had obsessively exercised to fight off unrest and agitation, as well as to render myself worthy of food, and relaxing was a foreign experience to me. I joined the gym she belonged to, and went there with her to work out in the water and to mellow out in the sauna and jacuzzi. I learned how to appreciate the way my body felt from doing those things. At the gym, I also asked for a program to help me build muscle as I put on weight. I didn't want to put on pounds and turn into the same shapeless blob I had been as an eleven year old, or else wind up with a dumpy, figureless body like my natural mother.

Tyanne also helped me learn to accept my larger body by going shopping for clothes with me. I had hated my body in or out of clothes since adolescence and did not know what looked good on me. I had worn boy's T-shirts and jeans for years; for dress-up, I wore mid-calf length skirts that made me look like I'd stepped out of the nineteenth century. Tyanne could walk into a clothing store and within minutes pick out complete outfits that I liked, that fit me, and that looked attractive on me. It was a talent of hers that I really admired; and, it helped me to overcome the conviction that I would always hate how I looked no matter what I wore. In time, I learned to *enjoy* wearing clothes and shopping for them.

The second part of my initial treatment contract was to learn to identify and to deal with feelings. I didn't even know what feelings were, so this was as big of a challenge to me as eating. My therapist, David, had me stand and physically push my arms against his (he was three times my size) to create an experience for me of frustration and anger. Although I was the only person in this center for emotionally disturbed adults with an eating disorder as a primary diagnosis, we all had in common a history of difficulty dealing with feelings. I looked to other students in the program for support and direction. We comprised a therapeutic community, and I had to get to know everyone else and let them get to know me. The support from the other students, and the friendships that I eventually made there, were invaluable to my recovery.

Therapy at Cathexis provided me with many experiences I had never had before. It was an extremely nurturing environment. On a daily basis, I asked for and received physical strokes. Part of the philosophy of the program was that our emotional problems were compounded by not having enough physical contact, so we asked for and gave a lot of shoulder and head rubs. Touching helped me to break down the barriers I had built to keep myself so alone with my unhappiness.

Regressive work gave me the opportunity to have a new experience of myself at a younger age and to superimpose healthy interactions on old childhood memories. During group therapy sessions, students contracted to be a specific younger age and were responded to accordingly. The results amazed me. For example, in role-playing a nine-month old baby, I crawled around exploring the room and returned when I wanted reassurance from my caretaker. No one chased after or hovered over me. If I started playing with a dangerous object, like a pencil, it was taken away and replaced with a toy; but, if I spilled water, I was allowed to get wet and play in the water. In a case like that during my actual childhood, I would have been immediately picked up and dried off. The overprotectiveness that had contributed to my fear of taking risks was supplanted with experiences in which I was allowed to learn about my own physical limitations.

During regressive work as an eighteen-month old, my contractual father, David, who was a very big man, tickled me and picked me up and turned me upside down as if I were a small child. I delighted in his warmth and strength and playfulness. From this work I experienced a new sense of trust, and also developed a sense of pleasure and self-acceptance about my body.

I also learned about being spontaneous and reactive to feelings, including hunger. My therapists reminded me that to a baby, hunger is a necessary and natural instinct, rather than a nuisance or a burden to caretakers. I cried when I was hungry or thirsty, and was fed. I ate with my fingers like a messy infant, and covered myself and the surroundings with food before the mess was cleaned up. I was not criticized for how dirty I had gotten myself or how much work I was causing my caretaker. My therapists stressed that babies are spontaneous and don't understand about being neat, clean, or well-behaved.

When I role-played a thirteen year old, I argued with my contractual parents about getting thin and dieting in a way I had never dared to seventeen years earlier when my anorexia first began. They allowed me to hassle, and responded to my fears of not being liked and of needing to look a certain way to be accepted.

As my weight approached the ominous 100 pound mark, I became increasingly anxious. When I reached 97 pounds, I tried to convince David that 98 pounds was a more appropriate goal for me and that I'd be healthier at that weight. The issue came up in a Nutrition Group meeting, and he was almost ready to let me stop gaining weight at 98 pounds. However, other people in the group who had personally experienced control struggles with therapists around weight themselves, argued that they did not think it was a good idea for me to stay under 100 pounds. To my chagrin, David ultimately agreed with them, and I reluctantly gained the additional weight.

The day I hit 100 pounds was not a joyous one for me. I was desperately unhappy because I no longer felt in control of that part of my life. This was their goal for me, and although I'd agreed to it, I had never wanted it. I was elated momentarily because I thought I could eat less food now, but I quickly became discouraged when I discovered that I would have to keep eating almost as much just to maintain my weight. Mostly I was overcome with feelings of loss and despair, and I had the same familiar anxieties about who I was and what was I going to do with myself. I thought that when I gained the weight, I would be cured, but instead I didn't feel much different inside. I was sure my therapists were wrong. Gaining the weight was nothing more than a deception. It hadn't made a difference. One evening in a treatment group I was very frightened and asked, "Now that I'm this person who weighs 100 pounds, who am I?" I felt completely empty inside. I was in tears and scared and felt fat and ugly. I said, "I gained all this weight the way I was supposed to, but I still feel the same, just fatter." My therapists reminded me of the other changes I had made in six months of treatment. I was beginning to identify and deal with feelings, and to form relationships with people in the program. They reassured me that developing interests to replace a food obsession was a process that would take some time, but that I was on my way.

I remember asking David how I could develop new interests if I wasn't even really sure what I did or didn't like. He inquired if I had heard a piece of music recently that I liked. I admitted that I had enjoyed listening to a recently released Steve Winwood album. He asked if I liked the music more the first time, or after hearing it several times. I thought about his question and replied that I liked it more after several listenings. David observed that the process of developing interests required my exposing myself to new things, giving myself a chance to become familiar with them, and then deciding whether or not I liked them. Whenever I became discouraged, it was David who asked if I was looking at a glass which was half empty or half full. He reminded me to look only at how far I had already come rather than how far I had left to go.

It took me at least two years to adjust to my body at normal weight; but eventually I stopped planning to lose the weight again after treatment. I was not happy with my new size, but I gradually began to accept it. In time, I came to believe that I would not be physically or emotionally healthy weighing any less than 100 pounds. If replaceable body parts were available, I might have chosen larger breasts, a smaller waist, and less proclivity to add weight to my hips. I would have liked to have been taller, too! However, I realized how similar my body shape was to my natural mother's, and that all the wishing in the world couldn't change genetics. All in all, though, I had not fared badly in the body lottery. I was aware of flaws in my own body, but I was no longer bothered by them. The significance of my body's shape and size was now far from first place on my list of priorities.

I've learned that being thin was a way for me to avoid being a sexual person. In the sexual relationships I had had with men in the past, it was not the sex I wanted, it was the nurturing, affection, and physical closeness. When I was a child, talking about sex in my household was prohibited, and I grew up believing that "sex is bad."

My mother disliked her body so much I couldn't imagine her liking sex. But my contractual mother's model was soft and feminine and she enjoyed being a woman. Tyanne and I had many long discussions about dating and men, just the kinds of talks I missed as a teenager. In time, I grew to understand that sex could be pleasurable and fun, and that I was in charge of my own sexuality.

In the process of being in treatment at Cathexis, I continued my quest for a career. For a long time I had wanted to be an artist because I loved being creative with color and texture, shape and form, but I didn't think I could make a living at it. I knew that I liked teaching and had enjoyed being a teaching assistant; but, I also knew that being a biology teacher was not for me. I wanted to teach people something about themselves, something they could use. I looked at both Tyanne and David, and saw the gratification they got from their work. Finally, I decided that I would combine the creativity and challenge of using different therapeutic techniques with my love of teaching and desire to help people by becoming a therapist. I had learned many skills from my own therapy, and I knew what had and had not worked for me. I believed that I could best make use of my experience by helping eating disordered persons, and I embarked on the most direct route to being a therapist in California, that of getting a Master's degree in psychology and a license as A Marriage, Family and Child Counselor.

For my Master's thesis, I wrote about anorexia nervosa. I included much of my personal history combined with research on information in the field. Originally, I only expected my thesis to be read by the few people on my Master's Committee. However, in 1983, my work was published as a book under the title *Dying to Please: Anorexia Nervosa and Its Cure.**

The Ongoing Process of Recovery

I stayed in treatment at Cathexis for about three years, tapering off from five to three days per week, three hours each day. After I graduated from the program, I remained in training there as I pursued my new career. Although Tyanne left Cathexis, I continued in therapy with her for another six years.

I knew that all that therapy had helped me in many ways. I had a support system of people who cared about me and to whom I could turn for help in solving problems. I wasn't isolated. I had internalized the things that I had been told and the processes I had been shown, and I was now able to care about myself and find ways to face my own problems. I was in a loving, supportive relation-

---

*Rumney, Avis; *Dying to Please: Anorexia Nervosa and Its Cure*; McFarland & Company, Inc. Publishers; 1983.

ship that my boyfriend, Rick, and I had both worked hard to build, I had several good friends, and a small but growing private practice. My work at Cathexis also helped to free me from old resentments I felt towards my parents. I stopped blaming them, as I once had, for modeling a course of unhappiness for me. I realized that they tried to be good parents and did the best job they could. I recognized the pain they experienced and even felt sad for them.

However, even after nine years of therapy, something was still missing. I expected that after all of those years of hard work, I would be happier and more at peace with myself. But I still felt empty when I wasn't busy or with someone who I knew cared a lot about me, and I didn't really feel secure about who I was.

I had always preferred doing to being, and viewed achievements as the measure of success and merit. This carried over to my practice as a therapist. I believed it was my responsibility to always provide my clients with the right answers to questions in their own lives. Once, when I had particular difficulty with a suicidal client, I sought the advice of a colleague and we ended up talking about me. She challenged me to look inward for what I was searching for outside, and I began to realize that I had been so caught up in my performance that I valued helping others more than I valued myself. By pursuing achievements, perfectionism, and other superficial values, I usually ended up dissatisfied. My colleague reminded me that I should be there for my client, but it was not up to me to take away her pain. She ultimately needed to look within herself for comfort, and so did I. My colleague also suggested that I try to be more accepting of myself and my own limitations; and, I left our meeting with new insight.

It seemed that my former quest for thinness was being replaced by a search for wholeness. My years in therapy had provided a solid foundation by showing me how to live and function in the world. I had learned how to get along better with other people, and through them to feel more comfortable with myself, but now I finally felt ready to learn how to live just with me. The real task was to accept whatever shortcomings I had and to trust in myself. A close friend of mine told me about some inspirational books she had been reading, and lent me some meditative literature. These exposed me to new ideas that were foreign to my upbringing and therapy. I found that reading this material often brought me a calmness reminiscent of walks on the beach or still moments gazing at the night sky. Unlike the escape I usually sought from books, reading this literature encouraged me to look inward. I had been so caught up in doing things that I rarely allowed myself time to be peaceful. I was too much of a workaholic to acknowledge my own needs.

I began to see that there was more to life than what I was pursuing. I appreciate that I've come a long way from where I was ten years ago: severely depressed, in a destructive relationship, weighing 70 pounds, and dancing topless for drunken sailors. My life is so different now. The external aspects are obviously improved, but more importantly, the inner parts are better, too. I now know that for me the attainment of self-acceptance and self-fulfillment is a process which is ongoing rather than a goal with a defineable end. I think that it's permissible to be working towards stilling the restlessness of my mind, though I do sometimes wish this endeavor wasn't so uncomfortable. I'm thankful to be finished with anorexia nervosa; my obsession with thinness is over forever. Walks on the beach, time spent with my boyfriend, meals with friends, and quiet moments bring me real pleasure. I now cherish time alone and try to free myself from my former obsession with undone tasks. It now seems natural to me that since ultimately, it is with myself that I must live, it is within myself that I must find my own completeness.

BULIMIA

About the Author

Lindsey Hall's secret obsession with food isolated her from family and friends, caused her health to deteriorate, and severely undercut her self-esteem. Food occupied all of her thoughts—even her dreams.

When she first wrote *Eat Without Fear* in 1980, there were no other publications available solely on bulimia, the binge-purge syndrome. It was a small booklet, which described her cure after nine years of overeating and vomiting four and five times daily. She expected the 100 copies that were printed to be a "final purge" and to leave bulimia behind; but, it has been reprinted about twenty times. It has been the inspiration for many people who have wanted to recover from their own eating disorders, and led Lindsey to become a pioneer in bulimia education and publishing. This newest, revised printing further describes the nature of her addiction, her healing process, and the personal progress she has made since her recovery.

She has been free from bulimia and food fears for more than ten years. She has received national recognition as a soft-sculpture artist, and loves being a wife, mother, businesswoman, and author.

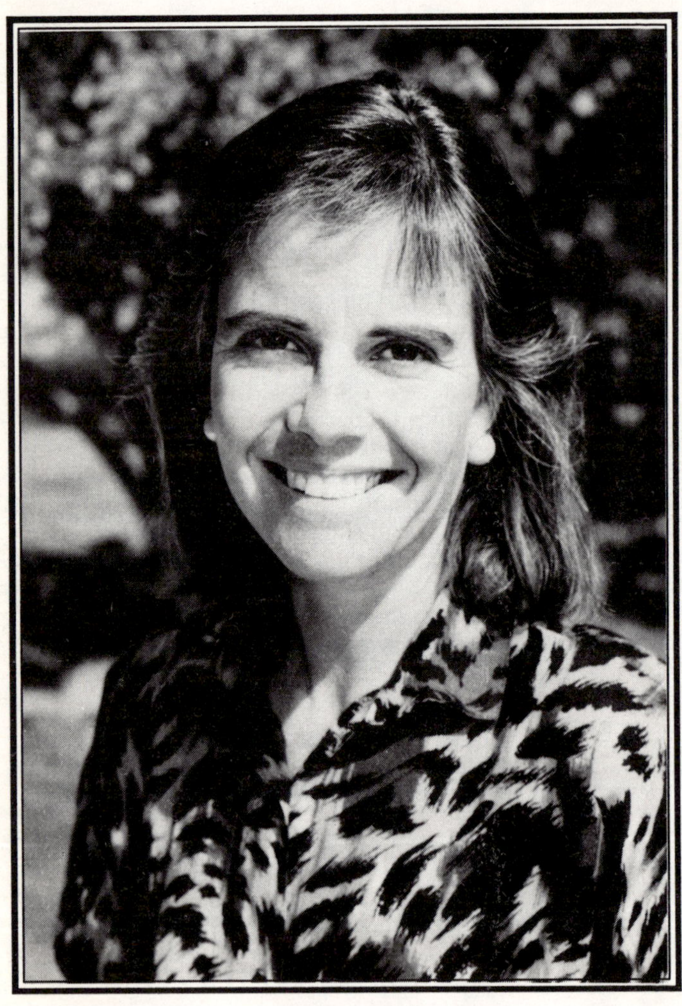

Lindsey Hall

Eat Without Fear

by

Lindsey Hall with Leigh Cohn

***

Introduction

I am wide awake and immediately out of bed. I think back to the night before when I made a new list of what I wanted to get done and how I wanted to be. My husband is not far behind me on his way into the bathroom to get ready for work. Maybe I can sneak onto the scale to see what I weigh this morning before he notices me. I am already in my private world. I feel overjoyed when the scale says that I stayed the same weight as I was the night before, and I can feel that slightly hungry feeling. Maybe IT will stop today, maybe today everything will change. What were the projects I was going to get done?

We eat the same breakfast, except that I take no butter on my toast, no cream in my coffee and never take seconds (until Doug gets out the door). Today I am going to be really good and that means eating certain predetermined portions of food and not taking one more bite than I think I am allowed. I am very careful to see that I don't take more than Doug. I judge by his body. I can feel the tension building. I wish Doug would hurry up and leave so I can get going!

As soon as he shuts the door, I try to get involved with one of the myriad of responsibilities on my list. I hate them all! I just want to crawl into a hole. I don't want to do anything. I'd rather eat. I am alone, I am nervous, I am no good, I always do everything wrong anyway, I am not in control, I can't make it through the day, I know it. It has been the same for so long.

I remember the starchy cereal I ate for breakfast. I am into the bathroom and onto the scale. It measures the same, BUT I DON'T WANT TO STAY THE SAME! I want to be thinner! I look in the mirror, I think my thighs are ugly and deformed looking. I see a lumpy, clumsy, pear-shaped wimp. There is always something wrong with what I see. I feel frustrated, trapped in this body, and I don't know what to do about it.

I float to the refrigerator knowing exactly what is there. I begin with last night's brownies. I always begin with the sweets. At first I try to make it look like nothing is missing, but my appetite is huge and I resolve to make another batch of brownies. I know there is half of a bag of cookies in the bathroom, hidden the night before, and I polish them off immediately. I take some milk so my vomiting will be smoother. I like the full feeling I get after downing a big glass. I get out six pieces of bread and toast one side in the broiler, turn them over and load them with patties of butter and put them under the broiler again until they are bubbling. I take all six pieces on a plate to the television and go back for a bowl of cereal and a banana to have along with them. Before the last toast is finished, I am already preparing the next batch of six more pieces. Maybe another brownie or five, and a couple of large bowls of ice cream, yogurt or cottage cheese. My stomach is stretched into a huge ball below my ribcage. I know I'll have to go into the bathroom soon, but I want to postpone it. I am in never-never land. I am waiting, feeling the pressure, pacing the floor in and out of the rooms. Time is passing. Time is passing. It is getting to be time.

I wander aimlessly through each of the rooms again, tidying, making the whole house neat and put back together. I finally make the turn into the bathroom. I brace my feet, pull my hair back and stick my finger down my throat, stroking twice, and get up a huge pile of food. Three times, four, and another pile of food. I can see everything come back. I am glad to see those brownies because they are SO fattening. The tension in my neck is easing, the pain is mixed with pleasure. The rhythm of the emptying is broken and my head is beginning to hurt. I stand up feeling dizzy, empty and weak. The whole episode has taken about an hour.

*****

For nine years, I binged and vomited up to four and five times daily. There were very few days without one binge, and thoughts of bingeing were always there, even in my dreams. It was painful and frightening. I do not binge anymore, but my healing was not an overnight thing. I worked hard and willingly, and underwent an amazing transformation! I am now free from bulimia and am healthy, happy, in love with my family, and successful as an artist, author, and businesswoman.

Beginning

I came from an affluent family that lived in a fancy home an hour north of New York City. My father commuted to the city where he worked as an investment banker. My mother was active in environmental causes, country club tennis, and amateur photography. I had three older siblings who paid little attention to me—except for one sister who teased me unmercifully. I was seven when the fifth child was born, and my parents hired a live-in couple to take care of me and my baby brother.

The overall impression I have of my childhood is of being alone and afraid that I had done something wrong. I didn't mean to get in trouble; on the contrary, I always tried to be a perfect little girl. Nevertheless, I had the perception that I was constantly screwing up, like the time I hid my brother's watch in cornstarch when he was chasing me, unaware of the damage that would be caused; or when I put my sister's toy animals in a pillowcase to show to someone, not realizing they were delicate china and would all break. My father made me suffer for that mistake! One of my biggest goof-ups was getting locked in my mother's clothes closet where I had gone to test a tie with a light on it. She went to New York, and I stayed locked away all day, crying and afraid. No one heard my screams, not the maid, the laundress, or my nanny. I was not found until my mother came home late that afternoon. Even though I was rescued, I felt like life in that house could go on without me and no one would notice. I was not the smartest, prettiest, oldest, youngest, or a boy, any of which, I thought, would have given me some importance in the household.

Most of the time, I retreated alone to my room, attic playroom, or the barns to play with the animals. I had a few friends who lived nearby, though I can't remember their coming to my house, and I avoided going to theirs for fear of their parents. One of the mothers used to laugh or yell at me when I didn't want to eat. Another threatened to hit me with a wooden spoon, and I was made to sit at the table until I finished. I was terrified of going there again—she made me eat tomatoes!

When I was ten years old at an annual physical exam, I thought I overheard the doctor tell my mother that I weighed too much. They said nothing to me, but after that I was conscious of my imperfect size. Salesgirls in the clothing store my mother took me to for dancing-school dresses always sympathized with my "figure problem" and recommended "A-line" skirts.

Despite my nickname, "Thunder Thighs," I wasn't obese. I weighed 142 pounds and was 5'6" tall. But I thought heavy legs and thighs were the most disgusting form of being overweight. Having a big chest still meant boys wanted to touch you, but being pear-shaped was an unspoken sin. I began to focus on my body as the source of my unhappiness. Every bite that went into my mouth was a naughty and selfish indulgence, and I became more and more disgusted with myself.

I went away to a prestigious East Coast boarding school at age fourteen. Everyone else from my grammar school class went away to private schools, too, as the local public school was considered "lower class." Without realizing how afraid I was or how to communicate my apprehensions, I left home in tears.

For months I cried at the slightest provocation. I had never approached my parents with problems and I had never confided in friends. I didn't even know what was bothering me. All I knew was that I was desperately unhappy.

The other girls at school all seemed beautiful and unapproachable: long fingernails, neat clothes, curly hair and THIN bodies. It was obvious that thin was "in" right from the start.

There were a few other girls whom I suspected had problems with food. One girl who roomed next to me for one quarter was always buying quarts of ice cream and hiding in her room. Then she would proudly announce that she was starting a diet which required fasting for the first two days. Another girl lost so much weight that her muscles could no longer hold up her 5'10" frame, and she walked bent over with her emaciated pelvis tucked forward for balance. She was taken out of school, rumored to have been throwing up all food in order to get skinny. That rumor was the first knowledge I had of someone forcibly vomiting. At that time, "bulimia" was unknown.

Even the other girl who attended the school from my home town decided to pull a "crazy" act by eating nothing but oranges for several months. I visited her in the infirmary where she had been sent for blood sugar tests because her weight was so low, and I didn't know what to say. I secretly envied her will power and her protruding ribs.

By the time I reached my senior year, my crying in public stopped, and I was no longer outwardly unhappy. I played sports, sang in the choir and had one good friend. She knew I thought of myself as ugly, and often reassured me that I was very pretty but I honestly thought she was humoring me like my parents did. I did my best to avoid situations which would make me feel like a failure. I begged to be let out of honors math, refused to be nominated for any offices, rarely went to dances, and was afraid to talk in class. I was happy to get cramps once a month and retreat to the safety of the infirmary. I didn't seek out many friends, and instead spent a lot of time alone or taking care of animals in the biology lab. I hoarded food in the dorm refrigerator and sometimes hid in my closet during dinner hour, sneaking food from my private stash. I kept a five pound can of peanut butter from which I snuck teaspoonsful during the days when no one was around. Thoughts of food were often with me although I had not yet binged and purged.

I constantly tried on clothes in front of a full-length mirror to see if they had gotten looser or tighter. I took up smoking cigarettes in private, which in my mind was a bad thing to do, but it was better than eating. I chewed gum, sometimes up to five packs a day. Through all this, I managed to hold my weight steady.

Then a friend went to a doctor who gave her a diet, and she lost ten pounds in one week. Playing down my desperation, I got my mother to take me to him. He gave me a pamphlet outlining the diet, and I returned to boarding school in the spring of my senior year thinking that I was really going to change. I was going to lose the extra twenty pounds that sat between me and happiness; but, the diet was horrible. I was weak and nauseous immediately. I was supposed to drink two tablespoonsful of vegetable oil before breakfast and dinner, eat only high protein foods, and drink 64 ounces of water daily. I lost eight pounds in one week, but felt bloated and nervous. Weak and sick, I went off the diet. I was a failure. At that time I had a boyfriend; but, when the diet failed, I quit seeing him. I also had the word "change" in two-foot letters cut out and pasted on one wall of my room, but I no longer expected that to happen. The last months of that year were extremely painful.

I started snooping in other girls' rooms to look at their belongings. I was on a clothing allowance and never felt that I could afford anything but essentials. I sometimes "stole" things, hoarding them for a few days or weeks until the newness wore off, and then I would try to return them, unnoticed. Often an item was reported lost and there was a big to-do about how low a person the thief must be, and I would have to maneuver the circumstances so it looked as if the victim had just misplaced the missing item. I didn't want to be thought of as a thief; I just wanted to be like everyone else for a short time.

The most devastating thoughts, though, were that other people could eat and I couldn't. I would watch the skinniest, most gorgeous girl spread brown sugar and butter on her toast every morning and never get fat—never seem to feel guilty! I was jealous of everyone who was thinner than I.

The first time I thought of sticking my fingers down my throat was during the last week of school, after I saw a girl come out of the bathroom with her face all red and her eyes puffy. She had always talked about her weight and how she should be dieting even though her body was really shapely. I knew instantly what she had just done.

I tried it three weeks later in a "Wimpyburger" stand overseas. I remember the secrecy, the pain of trying, and the excitement that I had found an answer to my prayers, I *could* be thin. I was spending the summer living with a Swedish farming family as an exchange student following graduation. I was afraid to decline food at any of their five daily meals! My weight got higher and higher because I couldn't always get all the food to come back up when I vomited. I was still experimenting. If a meal was dry and starchy, it would sit in my stomach and I would feel fat and bloated. During the summer, I tried to throw up at least once a day, often unsuccessfully, and left Sweden weighing 175 pounds.

I shocked everyone—including myself—by being accepted to Stanford University, 3,000 miles from home, and I left in a blatant show of independence and bravery. Once alone in my dorm room, however, I was faced with isolation and the hateful relationship I had with my Self. I retreated into eating which I knew would numb my anxiety, and I perfected the act of throwing up.

I began with breakfasts, which were served buffet-style on the main floor of the dorm. I learned which foods would come back up easily. When I woke in the morning, I often stuffed myself for half an hour and threw up before class. There were four stalls in the dorm bathroom, and I had to make sure no one caught me in the process. If it was too busy, I knew which restrooms on the way to class were likely to be empty. I always thought people noticed when I took huge portions at mealtimes, but I figured they assumed that I was an athlete and burned it off. Sometimes one meal did not satisfy the cravings, and I began to buy extra food. I always vowed that "this binge will be the last" and that I would magically and with ease metamorphose into a normal human being as soon as I threw up "this last time." I could eat a whole bag of cookies, half a dozen candy bars, and a quart of milk *on top of* a huge meal. Once a binge was under way, I did not stop until my stomach looked pregnant and I felt like I could not swallow one more time.

That year was the first of my nine years of obsessive eating and throwing up. I didn't want to tell anyone what I was doing, and I didn't want to stop. I was more attached to being numb than I was to anything else, and, although being in love or other distractions occasionally lessened the cravings, I always returned to the food.

I was convinced that bingeing was just a way to diet. There was nothing wrong with releasing tension by vomiting, even if I did it *everyday*, and I consumed tremendous quantities first. I did not consider myself addicted, and I could stop anytime, probably tomorrow.

My letters home fluctuated between questioning why I was at college and vague complaints about my health. Letter after letter said the same things: "I'm afraid, but don't worry about me." "I'm sick, but I'm being brave and getting better." "I'm probably going through some phase." Usually there was a tidbit of news at the end. With every plea for attention, there was quick reassurance that I didn't need it; and, as much as I wanted them to ask me about how alone I felt, I would have denied those feelings, I know it. I was a smart girl, had been to the best boarding school, came from a family of lawyers, bankers, and Ph.Ds. I was very athletic, seemingly independent and "together." How could I admit that I was throwing up my food to be thin?

Living with a Habit

I moved off campus in my second year because I couldn't stand the pressure of being around people all the time. I thought it looked like the kind of thing a liberated female would do, and no one questioned the move. I arranged my life to accommodate my habit, pretending to everyone, including myself, that I was being more of an adult. I vowed that when I got to the new place I would stop the eating and vomiting because I wouldn't have people around to make me nervous. I'd start an exercise program, become injected with will power, get thin, and the world would be mine. The only hitch was that as soon as I was alone, I started bingeing and throwing up again.

I decided what I really needed was a specific weight goal. When I got there I could stop feeling like I had to diet! I chose 110 pounds because I thought I'd probably look like a model at that weight. This goal stayed with me as an eight year obsession, and I only reached it for one day when I was dehydrated from vomiting. Even then it made no difference in my view of myself; I thought I looked the same—fat!

If I bicycled home from school, I usually carried cookies and doughnuts to eat as I pedalled. Sometimes I got home and threw up that batch only to be overwhelmed with tension an hour later, and I would set off again for an uphill ride to the grocery store. Then I could glide home downhill, cramming cookies in my mouth after the frantic, desperate ride up.

I always bought the same foods: one package of English muffins, a pound of real butter, usually a package of frozen doughnuts, a bag of Vienna finger cookies, and always milk (preferably chocolate) or ice cream—and maybe five or six candy bars to start off the binge. I would even eat waiting in line. I told the checkers that I was buying for a nursery school so they wouldn't suspect it was all for me. I could eat that much food in about an hour. If there was anything that I just couldn't finish, I threw it away, convinced and promising that this was the last time. If I hadn't bought enough food at the store, or if I was unable to get to the store at all, I would eat anything. It didn't matter. A couple of omelettes or a batch of sugar cookie dough, a loaf of toast or a whole cake.

It was different now that I was living alone. There was no worrying if the bathroom would be empty or if anyone would think it strange that I came into my room with a grocery bag full of the same foods every day. The addiction was in control.

One imagined problem—not having enough money—became a reality. My parents sent me tuition and an allowance, and I was in a work/study program testing mentally retarded children. I was happy about the work because it felt good to help others and it kept me away from food for a few hours at a time, but I always spent as much money as I earned.

It was at this point that I started stealing food. I felt a tremendous rush of independence and success when I got away with a bag of cookies or pound of butter. It was similar to my stealing at boarding school. I wanted what wasn't mine and what I felt was denied me. But there was one major difference: I did not plan on returning the goods. About six months later I was caught in a supermarket with a pint of substitute sugar in my purse, and the manager threatened me with jail. I promised to "go straight," and did, but the binges continued full force.

Marriage and a Secret Life

I had many short relationships that year which gave me attention, companionship, sex and fun, but not what I thought was love. Then Doug, who was a friend of a friend, began to visit me and I was overwhelmed by how much I liked being with him. As we spent more time together, I could tell that he was truly a good person. Ashamed, I decided not to tell Doug about my eating habits because I was sure that they would be changing "tomorrow" anyway. I was twenty and it felt nice to be in love. Our courtship, which lasted two years, was unavoidably spent apart much of the time. When we were together for intense weekends, I would be free from the food obsessions. As soon as I graduated from college and Doug was finished with his military service, we moved in together.

We opted to look for jobs on the East Coast and stayed in an apartment over my parents' garage while we were looking. My parents fell in love with Doug even though we were unmarried and sleeping together under their roof, which made me feel that I had made a good choice. As he was included in the family, I retreated. I was used to feeling unnoticed, and I filled that emotional hole with food. While everyone else had their own projects, I was on a direct road of eating and throwing up. I lived with them but felt like an outsider, sneaking my sandwiches and cookies, and throwing up in a bathroom with a loud fan so no one could hear what I was doing. Doug and I couldn't find jobs, and after six months we moved back to California where Doug was accepted to graduate school. We also decided to get married. I never expected my eating to be a negative influence on our marriage. I didn't think it would matter that my mind was usually elsewhere, dreaming about food, because I felt loved and in love.

Daily Life

For the five years I was married to Doug, the daily rituals and idiosyncrasies of my food problems became more and more rigid. I learned to put face powder on my eyes to hide the redness from the pressure of being upside down, and on my knuckles where they got raw from rubbing against my teeth. I routinely ran water in the sink to drown out the sounds of throwing up. I got on the scale every time I passed the bathroom as well as before and after every binge. I methodically tried on my clothes in front of a full-length mirror hoping they would hang looser than the time before. I became a meticulous housekeeper, especially when I did not have a job and was "working" at home. Sometimes I delayed throwing up while I vacuumed and washed dishes, eating all the time, to set the stage for the "cleaning" of my body.

One thing I had to do between binges was run back to the store to restock the food. There were days when I had to rebake batches of brownies a couple of times. I did dishes several times a day—I was averaging three to five binges everyday—and I was careful to check the toilet to be sure I'd left no traces. I hoarded bulk foods. I wanted everything to be orderly and clean in the closets and on bookshelves. *The only thing that was not just perfect was me!*

I was nervous in restaurants although we ate out a lot. For nine years I never ordered an entree because I wanted to look like I was dieting. Instead, I ordered a few side dishes, but I'd suggest we get ice cream after dinner to polish off the secret binge. I always ordered whole milk, because it was thick and smooth and made the food come up easier. I even knew which restaurants had private bathrooms.

Several times I came across a book or a person or a group which I thought had meaning for me. I clung to each of these for short periods of time, but any effects were not lasting. I read books on nutrition and health, thinking they would be a positive influence. To others I seemed like a health food freak. I took a course in anatomy and physiology because I thought that if I could see what I was doing to myself physically, maybe I would stop bingeing. I was always outside myself, separate from my behavior, wanting to control it.

I was surprisingly productive in those five years. I got my B.A. from Stanford University, held two challenging jobs, and did creative projects on my own. I started a business which is still running, and I kept up relationships with family and friends, albeit from a distance.

After nine years of bingeing, however, I began to have physical side effects, which worried me. My vision often became blurry and I had intense headaches. What used to be passing dizziness and weakness, after a few of my binges had become walking into doorjams and exhaustion. My complexion was poor and I was often constipated. I was usually dehydrated but didn't like to drink water because it made me feel bloated. Large blood blisters appeared in the back of my mouth from my fingernails. My teeth were a mess.

Still, I refused to see that I had a serious problem even though the signs were obvious: poor health, an increasingly distant marriage, isolation, low self-esteem, fits of depression, and secrets.

Shift in Focus

In spite of the intensity of my addiction, and that I kept it all secret, Doug and I did have many happy and loving times. We never questioned being together, but he was committed to many outside activities, and I had food. When Doug got an offer for a fellowship at Cornell University, we moved back to the East Coast. I was unable to find a job there, so I decided to experiment with a batik process I had learned.

For a year I crammed my artwork between binges. I had two private showings of the batik designs, which gave me enough positive reinforcement to continue. At the end of that year, I decided to take my batiks and some soft-sculpture dolls I had made to New York City for professional feedback. I planned to stay with relatives who I didn't know very well, which made me a little nervous, and I made appointments with designers. I tried to have confidence in my work and accept criticism willingly, but the pressure was tremendous. Several times, I stopped at a market to pick up huge stashes of food that I devoured in my room after everyone had gone to bed. One night, preoccupied by a binge, I left my papers where I had stopped for pizza and ice cream. I ran back through dark, unfamiliar New York City streets, oblivious to the danger. My food obsession had robbed me of rational thinking!

It was on this trip that I happened upon a magazine article about people who had problems similar to mine. The article was one of the first ever written about the bingeing and vomiting cycle, and the author considered it related to anorexia nervosa, an illness characterized by self starvation, but different because of the regular repetition of binges and purges. I was shocked! What's more, the author was conducting therapy groups five miles from where Doug and I lived!

My world suddenly shifted focus. I could not get the article out of my mind. When I returned home I spent a week bingeing heavily and then called the author, who told me to come right over. On my way, I stopped to stick my finger down my throat for what I was afraid would be the last time. What if she cured me today? I wasn't ready!

During the interview, I downplayed my lack of control and the severity of the problem. This was the first time I had told anyone! I don't know if the therapist guessed that I was holding back, but she invited me to join one of her ongoing therapy groups which would be meeting several days later. I told Doug that I had decided to deal with an old problem in a new way and added no details except that I was going for outside help. I stayed at home worrying that I would have to talk to a whole group of people about my binges.

When I got there, I presented my usual false front of confidence because I was scared to admit that I was an addict. I didn't want to say exactly how many binges a day I did, how much food I ate, how much time it took, or how alone I was most of the time—but I did. To say out loud, "I throw up five times a day," was extremely hard. The women in the group were very responsive and supportive even though each of them was struggling with her own issues. All along I had thought that I was the only person compulsively eating and vomiting, but the group helped me see that I was not alone. The therapist stressed the importance of taking actions such as speaking up, honestly acknowledging feelings, and keeping a journal. Sometimes I was able to put off binges for a day or two and I began to gain confidence that I would be able to continue getting better.

I stayed for five sessions, then Doug transferred back to Stanford. Recovering from bulimia was becoming my focus now, but I was still afraid to tell him anything. I decided that it would be a good idea for me to live alone for a while to concentrate on my cure. I told Doug that I would move to California too, but that I wanted my own place. I felt that we couldn't be together until *I had changed.* This was my addiction and I would return to him clean, pure, free, and independent when it was all behind me. He need never know.

When we got to California, we took separate places to live, which was painful and confusing for us both. We had never expected to be apart. Doug took an apartment in town, and I took a room in a house in the country. We saw each other daily, but it was always awkward. No matter what changes I felt inside, when we were together, I couldn't share them with him.

I liked Susan, the woman who owned the house where I lived, and I hoped that I could open up to her. But my bingeing began almost immediately, and I missed my group back in New York. I tried to keep up with my journal but was disgusted by my eating and wrote only about my daily life, not my feelings. Being around Stanford brought back many memories, and I returned to the same markets and doughnut shops that I used to frequent. Even though I had taken some daring steps towards curing myself, I still clung to the magical promise of getting better "tomorrow."

An art fair in Los Angeles was coming up in two months and I planned on selling my soft sculpture and batiks. I was hoping that it would be financially successful because my binges were expensive and I was running out of money. I kept on overeating and vomiting, assuming that when the fair came, things would change. I would make some money, spend some happy time with Doug, who was driving me, get some sun, and relax. I let my work on myself slide. Once again, my priority was not my cure, and I binged heavily until the fair.

Turning Point

I was really hopeful that the fair would be a turning point for me and it was, but not in a way I had expected. Monetarily it was a bust, and I sold practically nothing. By the end of the third day, I couldn't stand the thought of going back for the final day. I was a bundle of nerves and even broke down crying with Doug and his mother, with whom we were staying. I could not tell them that my greatest worries were about food, so they could not help me. I faced returning to the Bay Area to live alone, without a job, and unable to confide in anyone about the food problem that dominated my life.

It was not these aspects, though, that made the trip a turning point. It was meeting Leigh Cohn, a man who was also selling at the fair. I quickly felt close to him, and we spent hours talking when business was slow. I was conscious of his presence the entire time and did not want to say good-bye.

Within a week, Leigh and I exchanged letters and phone calls and made plans to see each other again. The attraction was incredibly strong. For three weeks, we spent almost every day together in what felt like a perfect union. Much to everyone's amazement, including our own, Leigh left an entire house of possessions in Los Angeles to live with me in my one room at Susan's so I could sell my dolls to contacts in the San Francisco Bay Area.

Doug reacted with disbelief, and we had many confrontations right from the start. My parents had been upset by our separation, but they found it incomprehensible that I was living with a man I had known for only a month. Even Susan disapproved. Everyone was against us.

Still, I felt on a very deep level that for once I was doing the right thing, and my Self blossomed in spite of the pressures. Unbelievably, the bulimia disappeared during those first weeks. Leigh and I were together almost constantly and the sudden difference in my daily routine felt wonderfully healthy and refreshing. This seemed to be that magical, instantaneous cure I had always wanted.

As the days started to follow a routine, however, my new-found strength began to fail me. I worried about the hurt I was causing my parents and Doug. I felt guilty for being so selfish. I began to question if I really was doing the right thing and if I knew my own mind! After all, I ate and vomited for nine years knowing full well I was doing something crazy; maybe I was still crazy.

As my tension increased, I began to sneak food while Leigh slept and when I was alone working at my studio. When I was bingeing, I felt numb and the doubts subsided, and I soon wanted to binge more and more. I could feel the desperation and loneliness building as it had in the past, and I was frustrated that being so completely in love hadn't completely cured me. I realized that I had a lot of work ahead if I was ever going to overcome my bulimia, and that if I didn't take the initiative then, I risked slipping permanently back into the addiction and would lose Leigh. I wanted all of my life to be as wonderful, loving, and free of bulimia as those first weeks together had been. I finally decided to take a chance and tell him, otherwise there was only secrecy and hiding. I wanted honesty and love.

The Healing Process

At first when I told Leigh about my bulimia, he thought it was not a serious problem. He had been a sweet-freak all his life, able to eat huge amounts of doughnuts and cookie dough without feeling guilty, gaining weight, or even getting cavities! He assumed that I was just a sweet-freak, too, and threw up because I felt guilty about it. As I described the size and the frequency of my binges, however, he could tell how desperate I was. It was a tearful, emotional outburst. He was compassionate, listened well, and resolved to help me.

I had always expected to get better *tomorrow*, but this time I knew that I had to start taking definite steps *now*. I made two resolutions. I would be absolutely honest and tell Leigh about all binges, and I would do anything to cure myself—even be locked away in a sanitarium or some unknown treatment facility if necessary. Leigh promised to stick by me as long as I stayed committed to my cure. He helped me come up with ideas about what actions I could take, listened, supported, laughed, and loved me; but we understood that I had to stop the bingeing by myself.

We made lists: immediate goals, future goals, what to do when alone instead of bingeing, things that were changing in my life, "Poor-Lindsey and Lucky-Lindsey" lists, what I liked and disliked about myself, how I felt about my parents, etc. I prepared a checklist of things I could do if I was on the verge of a binge. I did one item at a time until I overcame the desire to eat. Some of the diversions were to exercise, sew, garden, take a walk, or soak in a hot bath. The last thing on the list was to contact Leigh or another friend and talk about my feelings. I used this method about a dozen times and it worked well.

There were several new activities that I wanted to incorporate into my daily life. I didn't do all of these things every day, but I tried to be as consistent as possible. I began meditating regularly and started writing in my journal again. I tried to establish a positive frame of mind and feel more relaxed. I decided to drink a certain amount of water each day, but I had a hard time with that so I revised my expectations rather than feel like a failure. I also decided, at Leigh's suggestion, that I allow myself one "forbidden" treat daily without guilt. This was a completely different way to eat and surprisingly easy.

One major step I took, which is in the "junk food" category, requires a special preface. Although this activity had a tremendous impact on my confidence, to do it alone would have invited failure. No one should try this without support and supervision. Having said that, I'll describe an all-day binge I did with Leigh to prove that I didn't have to vomit. On the big day, I woke up to a bag of malted milk balls on the bedside table, which Leigh had gotten to start the binge *right!* We bought a pound of candy, a dozen doughnuts, caramel apples, caramel corn, a batch of homemade cookies, brownies and drinks—all to take with us in the car on a business trip we had to take to San Francisco. During the course of the day we also ate hamburgers and fries, milkshakes, a greasy meal of fish and chips, and an all-day-long continuous dessert of white chocolate. By bedtime, we were both exhausted and stuffed. Leigh felt sick, but I was preoccupied by how my body looked and felt. I looked pregnant and I couldn't lie down comfortably in any position. In spite of all this discomfort, I was actually quite proud of myself. I laughed at this incredible stunt I had accomplished. Leigh would not let me out of his sight for obvious reasons. I would never have tried this without a support person; undoubtedly, I would have vomited.

The next day we fasted, which was almost as frightening to me as it had been to binge the entire day before. But, after keeping in so much "junk food," I wanted my system to rest. Fasting turned out not to be as difficult as I had feared and I got hungry again by evening. I was sure I had gained weight, but I hadn't, and that made me even more confident. This was a real turning point for me—I knew I could reach a goal, and I had power over food.

I began reading books that I thought might help me learn more about my inner-self. I learned specific exercises I could do that enabled me to be more objective about some of my values and beliefs as well as my parents and childhood. I also read books about spiritual masters whose lives inspired me to be more loving towards myself and others.

When Leigh and I were first living together, I began to see a psychiatrist because of the tension and guilt I felt living with Leigh while still married to Doug. I didn't mention my bulimia at first, but when I did tell him, he recommended that I see a woman psychiatrist who had treated anorexics. At that time, bulimia was still virtually unknown by most people. I saw her once, but we did not relate well. I realized the importance of confiding in someone, however, and decided to continue using Leigh.

The most difficult thing that I had to do was to tell people the truth all the time. I started by sharing my bulimia with the people I least wanted to. Doug, who had finally accepted our separation as permanent, took my confiding as a genuine act of caring, and felt saddened by what I had been through. He was surprised and sympathetic; he said he didn't know why he hadn't asked me about why I was in the bathroom so much. I think we were closer after that than we had been in years.

About a month later, I substituted letter writing for journal entries. I always left open the option of not sending them or sending a revised copy. I wrote my parents letters that explained what I was going through, but did not ask for or expect much participation from them. I also talked to my brothers and sisters, who have confronted many of the same issues. Our conversations often gave me support because I was able to observe in them traits of my own, and they seemed okay!

I began to confide in friends. Most were interested, sympathetic and supportive, though a few dropped out of my life. I wrote the following in a letter to my childhood friend, the one who had eaten all those oranges at boarding school: "Finally I can tell people about eating and throwing up and not be ashamed. Do you know how ashamed I have been all these years, thinking I was abnormal and disgusting?"

Even when I wasn't bingeing, I was thinking about food most of the time, and this was very frustrating for me. I had a lot of pent up energy that I needed to release in ways other than bingeing. So Leigh and I wrestled on a large foam mattress on the floor and had exhausting fights with foam bats. I punched a boxing bag we had in our garage, and took long saunas. When I needed to, I screamed into a pillow until I was hoarse. All these things had a settling effect on my mind as well as my body.

During these months, I grew more comfortable with just being myself. I had always been desperate to maintain an image of unfailing perfection and independence, but now I stopped hiding my shyness, my anger, and my fears. Finally, as I grew to understand who I was and why, I also understood how well the bulimia had served me. It had been my friend, my buffer, my security, and my expression when I knew no other. As an addiction, however, it was allowing no other behavior but itself, and had taken me over. I fought hard to get me back!

The binges gradually diminished in number and size. During the first few months, I did several, but they dwindled to one every couple of months. When I did occasional binges, I considered them setbacks but used them to better understand why I binged and what I would do the next time to stop myself.

During the first six months of recovery, I pushed myself to do my program. Whatever were the causes for my bulimia—some I understood but others surely escaped me—my priority was living without it rather than trying to figure it out. Facing torturous cravings to binge and successfully replacing them had me on an emotional rollercoaster; but, little by little, the struggle got easier.

I Made It!

There came a point when days could go by without any thoughts of bingeing. I began to enjoy eating, cooking, and going to restaurants. After all of my perseverance, positive thinking had become more of a habit than a practice. At one point, I baked a cake for a couple of friends who were coming for dinner. They knew about my bulimia, and asked me how I could now make a cake without eating the whole thing. I told them that I forced myself to concentrate on the joy of the meal to come instead of feeling bad in any way. I wanted to be able to bake, just like anyone else, and it really wasn't that hard anymore.

My self-image was transforming. I began to think of myself as a funny, loving, successful, positive-minded person. If doubts crept up on me, I trusted that I was doing the right thing. Even being alone was enjoyable.

My social life underwent drastic changes. I made a conscious effort to resolve any conflicts left over from past relationships, and even rekindled some old friendships. In the past, I had made excuses to avoid being around people, but now I found that some of my happiest moments were with Leigh, my siblings, and friends. Although my parents did not actively participate in my recovery, they knew about it and did ask how I was doing. We became much closer. Doug and I divorced, but remained interested in and supportive of each other. I wasn't afraid of people anymore.

When business commitments ended in San Francisco, Leigh and I moved to Santa Barbara, away from the old haunts. We got married and continued to spend most of our time together. At first, a lot of our effort was spent on recovery; but, as that progressed, we focused more on my growing soft-sculpture business. We worked full-time with a staff, opened a retail store filled with my dolls, and expanded our wholesale market to more than 300 stores throughout the United States. I truly loved my life and respected who I had become.

A year and a half after I made the decision to stop, I considered myself "cured." Then Leigh and I wrote a pamphlet called *Eat Without Fear*, thinking that putting my bulimia on paper would be the final purge. My bingeing and vomiting were indeed over, but my involvement with eating disorders education was only beginning. I started getting letters from bulimics who were inspired to quit by *Eat Without Fear* . I was the first bulimic to talk about her own story on national television. Newspaper and magazine articles, some about me, began to appear. Public awareness about bulimia grew. We started giving lectures and workshops, wrote more about bulimia, and talked to many, many people who wanted to overcome their own food problems. We fell into an inspirational, educational role, which also became our business.

I'm gratified by the contributions I've made in this field, especially to those individuals who have been inspired by me to change. I certainly didn't expect to be in the role that I am, but since the start of my healing, little miracles have presented themselves; and, as I chose to notice them, they led me in this direction. I've followed my heart and gotten true nourishment—love.

CIGARETTE SMOKING

About the Author

Diane DuCharme estimates she smoked 169,700 cigarettes during a twelve-year period which began when she was a freshman in college.

At one point she quit smoking for three miserable years but never conquered the cravings. In 1975, she and her six-year old son struck a deal—he'd quit sucking his thumb if she'd quit smoking. This time she overcame her three-pack-a-day addiction through what she calls "The Cigarette Papers Plan."

She never smoked another cigarette and today is a happy non-smoker with rosy pink lungs. The founding Publisher/Editor-in-Chief of CompCare Publications in Minneapolis, Diane now lives in Northern California and is an advertising-public relations executive.

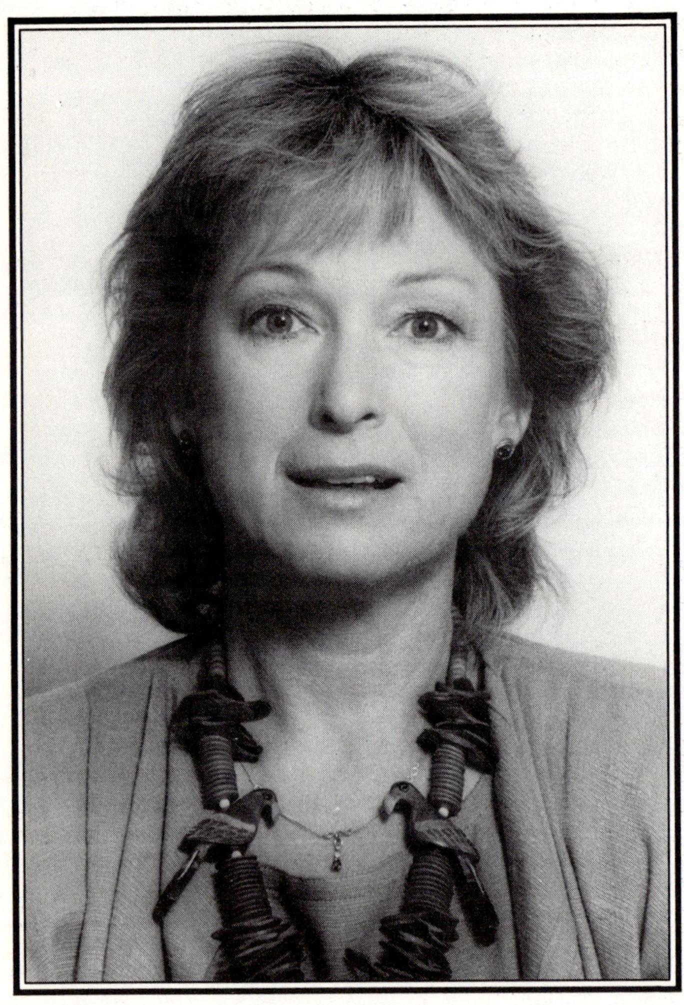

Diane DuCharme

The Cigarette Papers

by

Diane DuCharme

***

I Quit!

It now has been twelve years, six months, fourteen days and eight-odd hours since I ground out my last cigarette and crawled into bed, filled with fear, relief and determination to kick the habit permanently this time. Quitting smoking was no big deal. I wasn't addicted. Not very.

I'd smoked about 169,700 cigarettes over a twelve year period. I knew that continuing to smoke was an insidious slow form of suicide, sucking up energy and disposable income. Every cigarette I lit scarred my lungs just a little more and moved me one step closer to emphysema, cancer, heart disease, and a variety of other ills. I'd tried to quit several times before, once for almost three years. Yet for years I still harbored a little glimmer of hope that I could somehow hang onto my cigarettes and live the way all those women smokers in magazine ads and movies seemed to live. I consoled myself by thinking that at least smoking kept me thinner, making it possible to keep my weight at about 115 pounds.

I'd look at the women in the cigarette ads and wonder why the illusion *never* matched my realities. These women always are fine physical specimens who wear perfectly-fitted white tennis dresses (no pocket bulges where the cigarettes and lighters are stuffed). They are always photographed standing around the court, grinning and juggling their tennis racquets and their cigarettes. First of all, I could never gracefully hold both a tennis racquet and a cigarette at the same time. And secondly, when *I* stood around the court, I was red-of-face, huffing and wheezing, because my lungs were killing me.

Or beautiful svelte smokers are pictured at elegant parties and the theater in $2,000 designer gowns. In those scenes they never drop ashes on the host's carpet, never burn their designer dresses, never have trouble balancing food, drink AND a cigarette while standing in a shoulder-to-shoulder crowd (and who, may I ask, is holding their purses?), never have to flee the theater with a coughing fit during a dramatic moment—and never have to frantically fan away the cigarette smoke curling into a companion's face during an intimate discussion. Most wonderful of all, the ashtrays are never filled with cold, smelly ashes or lipstick-stained butts.

Where are the ads which show a woman so frantic for a smoke that she is driving 15 minutes out of the way in rush hour traffic to buy cigarettes and/or matches before going to work? Or almost crashing into another car on the freeway while retrieving a dropped, lit cigarette on the floor? Or leaving her small sleeping child alone at midnight on a blizzardy Minnesota night to find an open 7-11 store? Or shaking the change out of her son's piggy bank because she was out of both change and cigarettes?

Just Like Any Other Addiction

I didn't admit to myself just how addicted I was and how crazy my behavior was until I became managing editor of Hazelden Publications in 1974 and began working with members of Twelve Step organizations such as Alcoholics Anonymous, Alanon, and Overeaters Anonymous. The behavioral parallels to food addictions or alcohol/drug addictions were obvious, even to a slow learner like me. For example:

* *One cigarette was too much, and a thousand were not enough.* During my last few years of smoking, I was inhaling about three packs a day. Sixty cigarettes. I figure I was awake about 17 hours a day after deducting time for sleeping and showering: that comes out to about three cigarettes an hour. I even kept them on my night stand for times when I woke up during the night. I frequently promised myself, with little success, that I'd cut back, ration them out.

* *Protecting my "stash" was vital.* Before I left the house, I'd calculate the number of cigarettes and matches I'd need to get me through an event, worry whether I'd be able to buy them where I was going, whether I had plenty for the trip. Before I went home, I'd calculate again whether I had enough to get me through the night. I knew this kind of planning took time and effort which could have been put to better use!

* *I spent money on cigarettes which should have been earmarked for other things.* Maybe by comparison, cocaine and heroin addicts consider the cost of cigarettes a mere pittance, but to many average Americans, paying for more than 1,000 packs of

cigarettes a year takes a significant chunk of disposable income while returning no benefits. I was divorced when Philip, my son, was only three. For the first few years money was a scarce commodity, to put it mildly. I may have postponed getting my teeth cleaned or my rundown heels repaired, but somehow I always found enough money for cigarettes, even when the consumption climbed from one pack to two to three and the costs skyrocketed.

* *I denied how much I smoked and how it affected my life.* I never told anyone how many cigarettes I actually smoked and how dependent I was. I rarely wrote a memo or made a phone call without a cigarette in my hand. Although the phrase "secondhand smoke" had not yet been coined, I knew it wasn't a good sign when I snuggled Philip and smelled my cigarette smoke on his clothes and in his hair. I told others (and myself) that I suffered from frequently recurring bronchitis and an allergy to my mascara without considering that smoking might be the cause.

* *I kept promising myself that I'd cut back—but I couldn't.* During the last three years that I smoked (after breaking three years of abstinence) I'd give myself a little pep talk almost every morning, "OK, Diane, today is going to be different. You won't light a cigarette until you get to the office. And you'll only have one an hour during the day. And only one after dinner. You can do it!" Most nights I fell into bed once again with aching lungs and smelly fingers. I felt like a failure because my willpower wasn't strong enough to wean me away from my addiction which I wanted so badly to shake. On those rare days I *did* stick to my plan, I'd often reward myself with extra cigarettes that evening. Just your standard, basic addictive behavior.

* *In my lucid moments I was disgusted with myself.* In another parallel to chemical dependency, I was getting sick and tired of being sick and tired. My fingers stunk. My breath was always bad, no matter how many times I brushed my teeth and how many breath mints I devoured. At the age of thirty I was in lousy physical condition. It hurt to even think about running or skiing or hiking or biking. I coughed when I climbed several flights of stairs. But I couldn't envision living any other way. Three years of constant cravings had driven me back to the cigarettes after my last abortive attempt to become a nonsmoker.

* *My favorite companions were other smokers.* They didn't criticize me. They smelled just as badly as I did. And they usually had cigarettes to lend me when I ran out. We could sit around for hours, drinking coffee and enjoying our conversations with very rare mention of our mutual addictions. If the smoke blew in your face, you just wafted it away. You didn't have to worry about offending anyone. We all agreed that our *least* favorite companions were ex-smokers.

* *People who cared about me confronted me about my smoking habit.* One of my first post-college jobs was that of program-publicity director for the Greater Minneapolis Heart Association. My tasks included introducing Heart Association films to civic and educational groups, and organizing and arranging a metropolitan area series of cardiopulmonary resuscitation training programs for hospitals, fire departments and police departments. I worked closely with a young doctor who actually taught the classes. After several months he looked at me in disgust and said, "How can you be in there talking about taking care of your heart and then come out in the corridor and light up a cigarette? I'm almost ashamed to be on the same program with you." I felt both guilty and defensive. After all, it was my body and my health and I could do as I pleased, couldn't I? I finally admitted he was right but said I *liked* my cigarettes and *liked* smoking. As a compromise, I did all my smoking outside after that.

Several years later my mother was hospitalized for surgery and shared a room with a woman, a heavy smoker for many years, who was dying of lung cancer. The woman herself begged me to quit smoking while I was still young, before it was too late. I looked at her lying there, tried to imagine what it would be like to switch bodies with her, and got very nauseated. I rushed out to the waiting room and yanked a cigarette out of my purse to soothe my discomfort.

A few years after that my son started learning in nursery school and on Sesame Street about the nasty effects of smoking on health. From then on, every time he saw me light up, he'd run to me crying, "Mommy, Mommy, don't. You'll kill yourself." I tried not to smoke in the house unless he was outside or asleep, but I still couldn't quit. I felt just as rotten about terrifying him as I did about my inability to drop a habit which caused me more grief than pleasure.

I Still Wanted to Smoke . . .

It was all very puzzling to me. I started smoking when I was 18 because I wanted to look older, be more sophisticated, rebel against my parents. No one talked then about connections between nicotine and health problems. Now I was over 30, knew thousands of reasons not to smoke and was intellectually convinced that I wanted to quit, to be free of cigarettes and everything they represented. Emotionally, though, I hadn't been able to disconnect myself from my habit.

I *did* still enjoy that first cigarette in the morning with a cup of fresh coffee. And the one after dinner. And the one after . . . sex, as made famous by the likes of Bogie and Bacall. I was (am) sometimes shy, and smoking gave me something to do with my hands at parties and meetings.

The whole ritual of cigarette smoking is invaluable when you are embroiled in disagreement: "I'm very angry with you." (Removal of cigarette from package and tap-tap on table.) "I think you're acting like a child." (Insert cigarette in mouth, narrow down eyes into slits, take deep breath through nose.) "I can't imagine where you ever got that idea." (Disdainful sideways glance as you strike match and bring it to cigarette.) "I never would have promised *that!*" (First deep inhalation as you try to look like Kathryn Hepburn) . . . "Don't . . . ever . . . say . . . that . . . to . . . me . . . again." (Exhalation of dense fog of smoke which separates you from opponent.) As a matter of fact, I never have found an adequate substitute prop for such scenes.

. . . But I Wanted to Quit Even More

My reasons for wanting to quit far outweighed my reasons to continue. First and foremost was the terror that I knew my smoking caused Philip, and my fear about how the second-hand smoke affected him. He suffered from frequent sore throats and colds, especially during locked-in, closed-up Minnesota winters when there was no fresh air in the house. My survey may have been unscientific, but it was quite obvious to me that my nonsmoking friends' children suffered fewer bronchial problems than my own son or children of my smoking friends.

I was worried about my health, my coughing, my shortness of breath. There was nothing cute about having foul breath and stained fingers. My vanity got the best of me when I read that women who smoke wrinkle earlier and more severely than women who don't. (I may have ample thighs—but God gave me great skin which partially compensates on the divine balance scale of credits and debits!)

The amount of money I burned up every year while buying cigarettes, repairing singed spots on my clothing, and making frequent trips to the dry cleaner was no small factor. I would rather have spent it on clothing or vacations for Phil and me.

As the number of ex- and nonsmokers swelled and more scientific evidence linked smoking with disease, a growing number of people in restaurants, offices and parties didn't want you smoking near them. It wasn't fun to feel forced to jostle through the crowds into the lobby during concert and theater intermissions. More and more often I felt like an outcast, rather than like "one of the gang."

My list of reasons not to smoke grew longer and longer, but I still couldn't summon up enough willpower to quit. One night as I was lying in bed, counting up the day's tobacco consumption and sniffing my nasty fingers, I had a great revelation : I didn't have to 100% want to give up smoking before I could do it. I just had to 51% want not to smoke—in other words, want *not* to smoke more badly than I *wanted* to smoke. Aha.

The next problem was figuring out when and how to quit forever without duplicating the miseries I'd suffered during my previous three-year stretch of abstinence. I didn't feel I could attend any classes offered by the American Cancer Society or join any private programs such as Smokenders, although I'd read all their materials and knew their philosophies. I was driving 100 miles a day round trip to work. That, plus my business trips and my responsibilities as a single parent, left no time for a formal structured program.

Seven years earlier I managed to quit (for a three-year period) because my then-husband (a smoker) and I wanted to have a baby. I quit cold turkey, just quit without making a plan, and substituted countless rolls of peppermint Lifesavers for the cigarettes. In one month I added 20 pounds to my 5'3" frame. I was miserable and craved cigarettes all the time. The next month I went off the pill. The third month I got pregnant, and the major league weight gain began. I waddled into the delivery room weighing 173 pounds and gave birth to my six-pound Philip. I waddled out of the hospital weighing 161 pounds instead of my "normal" 115 pounds. I was wearing a size 13 maternity dress, and it was tight.

During those three years I was what Alcoholics Anonymous members would have described as a "dry drunk." I never touched a cigarette, but I wanted to. I thought about it frequently and felt deprived. I didn't have any terrific substitute ways for coping with stress or rewarding myself. I'd inhale smoke drifting by me from my husband's cigarette. I felt fat and unhappy because I couldn't get rid of the last ten to fifteen pounds of post-baby flab and wear all my old clothes.

One day my husband asked me to light him a cigarette while he was driving. Would I? Wowee. It may have been thoughtless on his part because he knew what a struggle I was having with my self-control, but it was the only excuse I needed! I did it again and again. One day I bought my own pack, theoretically because I didn't like his brand. I rationalized that I would just smoke until I lost fifteen pounds and quit again.

I lost the weight, but all of a sudden I was in the midst of a divorce and rationalized that I needed to keep smoking to deal with the stress. Three years later the stress had not lessened, but my daily smoking intake had doubled and then tripled to 60 cigarettes, seven days a week, without pause. It was almost as though my addicted body was compensating for the three years it had been forced to go without nicotine.

Making the "Cigarette Papers" Plan

Those experiences were still very vivid. This time I knew I would have to handle things differently if I was going to quit smoking permanently and comfortably. I decided to pour my years of reading, research, and experience into a personal plan (which I dubbed "The Cigarette Papers") rather than randomly throwing away my cigarette pack. I knew enough now about Twelve Step programs to know that I'd have to use the "One Day at a Time" approach. And I knew enough about myself to know that I'd have to totally break my familiar patterns long enough to get the cigarettes out of my life. A third key element was figuring out new ways to reward myself, comfort myself, energize myself.

I wasn't anywhere near ready to quit when Phil, whose conception was the impetus for my first attempt at quitting, once again propelled me into action. At age six, he still was sucking his thumb and carrying everywhere a filthy little ball of satin and fuzz which once had been "the cuddle blanket." With all my motherly wisdom, I begged and wheedled and told him what a big boy he was. I knew he didn't need to suck his thumb anymore. He looked at me thoughtfully and said, "How come, Mom, it's okay for you to smoke but it's not okay for me to suck my thumb?"

Crash of cymbals. Bolts of lightning. The kid was right, once again!!!

"Good point, Phil," I said. "Good point."

We made a deal and shook on it. I would quit if he would quit. He handed over the corpse of the blanket.

It was New Year's Eve, theoretically the ideal time for new beginnings and action on The Cigarette Papers Plan. It wasn't the leisurely transition I'd intended but it did give me four days of grace before facing the office routine of long commutes, long meetings, long hours on the phone, long hours in front of a typewriter keyboard writing and editing, all of which lent themselves so well to smoking.

Phil was spending several days with his father. I already had plans to spend the holiday time with favorite former Minneapolis friends (intermittent smokers with whom I had shared many packs!) now living in Chicago but visiting Minnesota. Both husband and wife were in a nonsmoking mode at the time—and were delighted to support my crash plan. Their first great idea was to take the train rather than fly to Chicago. I'd be locked on the train for about eleven hours with no access to cigarettes but with lots of fresh fruit, soft drinks, magazines, and conversation. Sounded good to me.

Before we left Minneapolis, I made an appointment to have my teeth cleaned on the day I returned, something I've recommended ever since to neophyte stop-smokers.

The train trip was a new experience and a treat for me.

During my stay in Chicago, my friend Sina taught me the rudiments of scarf-knitting which kept my hands busy when they wanted to fondle cigarettes. I had fun and felt pampered. Every time I craved a cigarette, I reviewed my list of reasons to quit smoking and visualized Phil's solemn little face as we made our "deal." I prayed a lot, gulped deep breaths, went for lots of walks, drank gallons of juice, took frequent baths and showers, muttered "A day at a time" every minute or so—and proudly flew back to Minneapolis, knitting away in the nonsmoking section. Physically, I was still suffering withdrawal pains (for example, headaches and insomnia) but I felt triumphant.

I told myself that I wasn't quitting forever, just until my seventy-fifth birthday.

Psychologically, I was in a better spot. In contrast to the first time I quit, I immediately began enjoying my gains of freedom and health and money rather than mourning the loss of my friend, tobacco. That made the difference. I began to notice for the first time how many people *didn't* smoke rather than how many did.

Before I went back to work, I finalized my plan for coping with my tobacco cravings. During the months that I had been developing The Cigarette Papers Plan, I wrote pages and pages in notebooks about why I smoked, why I wanted to quit, times I craved them the most, other ways I could take care of myself, inspirational quotes, prayers, and introspective little essays. I edited it down to the key elements and transferred The Plan onto index cards which I kept just as near to me as I used to keep my cigarettes.

Selecting the right substitute for my oral fix and my need to have something to hold and play with was a challenge. Lifesavers were not the answer! At least I'd learned that much the first time. Sugarless gum was a help, but when I'm absent-mindedly chewing gum, I resemble a cud-chewing cow. I settled on cinnamon sticks—no calories, bitter but tasty, easy to carry. Some days I chewed so many cinnamon sticks that my tongue burned. I've never met anyone else who thought this was even a moderately good idea, but it worked for me.

Early morning prayer and meditation were essential for me. I read one or more Twelve Step daily meditation books as part of my serenity program. I learned more visualization and centering techniques. I talked each day with at least one person who was on a Twelve Step Program, an easy assignment because I was working at Hazelden. I attended various Twelve Step Program meetings with friends—AA, Alanon, Overeaters Anonymous, it didn't matter which. I always came away feeling more centered and stronger.

Whenever I was most sorely tempted, I whipped out a little notebook and jotted down the circumstances and time of day. This served two purposes—it occupied me for a few minutes and also helped me to be wary whenever a similar situation occurred. If I still felt obsessed when I'd finished writing, I'd take a few deliberate deep breaths (sometimes so deep that people walking by my office thought I was hyperventilating!). If the craving was still relentless, I'd take a brisk five-minute walk. Usually that got me through the crisis.

I avoided smokers for the first few weeks just as diligently as I formerly sought them out. I tried to hang around with people who were also reformed cigarette smokers and would give me lots of positive strokes. Incidentally, most of those who had first given up alcohol and then smoking found quitting smoking to be the tougher of the two. Most experts advise avoiding beverages which you commonly paired with your cigarettes (such as alcohol and coffee) for the first month or so. Giving up alcohol was no big deal, but I decided going cold turkey on my coffee AND my cigarettes was more deprivation than I wished, thank you. I had always drunk coffee strong and black, so I added milk to it to disassociate it from my smoking patterns. I personally never pinpointed a time when drinking coffee set off severe cigarette cravings.

I asked every former smoker I met for hints and supportive ideas and tried out most of them. One idea I loved, but rejected anyway, was that I plant ivy in my car ashtray. I did seriously consider it for a few days.

Phil had a much easier time of it than I did. He missed the blanket for about two nights and then thought, "Wow. I'm grown up. I don't need to suck my thumb any more!" We congratulated each other frequently and celebrated our successes. That was the sweetest part of all!

Changing My Life

I was hungrier. I did gain back those fifteen pounds, even though I exercised more and paid attention to the quantity and quality of my meals. I began to get suspicions, later confirmed by the Surgeon General's Report, that nicotine does affect one's rate of metabolism. Most of the time I didn't let myself substitute snacks for cigarettes (remember the nasty cinnamon sticks). I noticed how the tobacco companies focus on women's fears of weight gain in the way they market cigarettes, even with the names, such as "Virginia Slims," and the long, sleek shapes. This time I didn't buy into that fear. My long-term gains were worth a few pounds.

I scheduled regular rewards for Phil and me—outings, movies, facials, new makeup, lunches with favorite friends. At first I allotted us the equivalent funds I had been spending on tobacco—it would just have been burned up anyway, so I regarded it as an investment in our health and happiness.

Frequently during the first few months, my stress levels shot up so high that I didn't see how I could possibly make it through one more day without a cigarette. I was in an intense, high-pressure job with long hours, many of them spent alone in a car, some of them spent alone in hotel rooms. For twelve years, I had smoked during tough phone calls, while I was writing papers and articles, when I was staying up working until two A.M., when a relationship fell apart, when I was lonely. Whatever the situation, grabbing a cigarette bought me time to think. The nicotine kept me awake and functioning when I was exhausted. Smoking had become such an automatic reflex action that sometimes my brain cells felt they would never kick in again until I lit them a cigarette. Gradually, but slowly, my new coping mechanisms—the pause for serenity, the deep breathing, the brisk walk—replaced the cigarettes.

The first time I quit smoking I wasn't acutely aware of the process because I was soon pregnant and absorbed with that. This time I noticed. The physical withdrawal pains were uncomfortable for the first several weeks. My skin broke out with rashes, boils, and pimples on my face and body. As a matter of fact, the first few months were hell. I kept coughing up crud from my lungs. I felt depressed and cried easily. I had headaches. The second three months were moderately dreadful. At one point I decided I just couldn't go any longer without a relapse. That night I went to an Overeaters Anonymous meeting in my neighborhood. I looked around the table at all the overweight women with cigarette packages in front of them—and decided smoking wouldn't make anything better.

That seemed to be a turning point. The next day I felt better, and the cravings began to recede permanently. Almost a year passed before I quit thinking about how good that smoke felt rushing into my lungs and started thinking instead about how noxious it felt to have it blown in my face by someone still smoking.

I was startled to wake up from a most realistic dream, 3-D and in color, a full five years after my last cigarette. I dreamt I was smoking. I could feel it, taste it, smell it. I felt horrible because I had blown it. Oh God, I thought, now I'm going to have to go through withdrawal again. I can't quit smoking all over again. It took me several minutes to realize that this hadn't happened. The dream recurred several times, but never so vividly. I have read since that this is not an uncommon reaction for ex-smokers, especially at times when faced by difficult circumstances and decisions.

Working Through the Four Stages of Quitting

From my own experiences and that of friends, I believe you can't just toss away the cigarettes and skip from being a smoker to being a non-smoker. It's a four-stage process—and if you get stuck at any of the interim stages, you'll probably return to smoking. Here is how I define them:

1) *The Smoker:* Obvious.

2) *The Smoker Who is Not Currently Smoking:* The stage I was stuck at the first time I quit. The nicotine addict's version of a dry drunk. Secondhand smoke still smells good.

3) *The Ex-Smoker or Former Smoker*: Severe cravings have passed but the wistful memories linger of just how good that cigarette tasted with the first cup of breakfast coffee. Links with the world of smokers not totally broken.

4) *The Non-Smoker*: The lungs are pink and rosy again! It's difficult to remain objective and friendly when a smoker sits next to you in a restaurant or blows smoke in your face. Friends who didn't know you in your puffing days are astounded to learn that you once had the habit. As a matter of fact, it's so far from your daily consciousness that you're a little astounded yourself when you think about it. For example, instead of looking forward to resuming smoking on my seventy-fifth birthday, I'm planning to take a camping trip into the Sierras.

Breaking my smoking addiction was the first step to completely changing my lifestyle. I'm over forty now, and far healthier than I was twelve years ago. Three years ago I ran the Bay to Breakers, a 7.5 mile San Francisco race. I regularly hike, ski, dance, go camping and work out. I still can't ride a bicycle, but that's because I fall over when I make left turns.

Although I probably would be thinner if I smoked today, I'd never trade the poundage for the coughs, chest constrictions, bad breath, stained teeth and fingers, and wrinkles that come with the cigarettes. Thanks to my lousy metabolism, I slide twenty pounds up and down the scale, depending upon my stress levels and the amount of exercise I'm getting. About seven years ago I got down to 110 pounds and was able to stay there by rigidly eating 600-1,200 calories a day and working out 12 to 14 hours a week. That kind of regimen seemed as unrewarding as smoking! Now I'm concentrating on health, on being more accepting of my body type. I keep my calorie intake to about 1,200 to 1,500 calories a day, and work out five to seven hours per week. And I feel *great*.

Phil is now eighteen and has completed his first two quarters of college at the University of Minnesota. He has never (and says he will never) smoked a single cigarette. For that I am proud and grateful.

What I've Learned Since I Quit

In the twelve years since I quit smoking, science and technology have marched on. I now know many things I wish I had known then but which I try to share with friends and acquaintances who are still trying to unhook from their nicotine addiction.

In 1964 when the first U.S. Surgeon General's Report on Smoking and Health was issued, about 53% of U.S. adult men and 32% of the women smoked. By 1986 only 29.5% of the men and 23.8% of the women smoked.

Dr. Ron Davis, who directs the U.S. Office on Smoking and Health, said, "I believe that people are now beginning to realize that smoking is not just a minor health hazard. It's actually the most important preventable cause of death in our society."

It's worth it for smokers to use every help they can get in their attempts to break the habit. New helps are appearing regularly. For example, I've just read about a project financed by grants from the National Heart, Lung and Blood Institute (part of the Department of Health and Human Services). Called "The StopSmoking System," it connects a smoker with a personal computer and modem to a 24-hour-a-day electronic counselor via CompuServe. The "counselor" is programmed to respond to smokers learning to quit. Through the modem, the new ex-smoker can communicate with others who are trying to quit. I like that idea.

I read the Surgeon General's Report on Smoking about ten years ago, and was relieved to learn that many of my hunches have been substantiated about what happens physically while we are becoming nonsmokers. Surprisingly, the information about cancer, lung disease, and heart disease has been disseminated widely but I've rarely seen anything reported about the effects on skin and metabolism during the nicotine withdrawal period.

I suffered severe skin problems for the first few months after I quit, although I had never suffered from skin problems before. Somehow I thought it must be related to stopping smoking, but I couldn't find any research which mentioned this side-effect. The woman who gave me facials told me that other customers frequently suffered the same symptoms after they quit, but she, too, couldn't corroborate this with any scientific evidence. There it was in the Surgeon General's Report—the toxic substances such as gases and poisons deposited in the body from smoking did indeed work their way out of the system through the lungs and the skin. (And they took their sweet time about it.)

When someone quits smoking, their metabolism will change, at least temporarily. The standard wisdom in 1975 when I quit was that the only reason one gained weight after dumping the cigarettes was that one was eating more as a substitute or because the food tasted better. I knew that couldn't be true because I wasn't eating any more the second time I quit and may even have been eating less. No one believed me.

Indeed, the Surgeon General's Report validated that nicotine speeds up metabolism, in addition to speeding up the heart rate. Ergo, removal of nicotine slows down the metabolism. To remain at the same weight, one must cut back on food quantities and exercise more.

After plowing through hundreds of heavy scholarly pages in the Surgeon General's Report about cancer, pregnancy problems, heart disease, etc., I was delighted to find a research study which made me laugh out loud, although I still don't understand its significance. It seems some university divided their research rats into two groups, gave nicotine to one group, and then made both groups swim. Their findings: the rats who got the nicotine swam less than the other group. I had visions of all these rats wearing bikinis and sunglasses, lying around a swimming pool, painting their toenails red, and puffing on Virginia Slims.

So what do I tell the people I know who are trying to quit? Don't wait for the perfect time to quit. It will never come. Make a personal plan, just as I did. Investigate all the classes and groups in your community such as those offered by the American Cancer Society, the Lung Association, Smokenders. Check out organizations such as Schick which have in-patient therapy. Get to know people in Twelve Step Programs such as Alcoholics Anonymous, Overeaters Anonymous, or Alanon. They have a beautiful philosophy which will help you, whatever your addiction, and members are happy to share the philosophy with you. Then decide which helps feel right for you.

Write down your plan, including the benefits you will gain and the ways you will reward yourself. Exercise is extremely important; write down the ways and times you will get yours. List the crutches you will lean on when you most desperately want a cigarette—and let me know if you plant ivy in your car ashtray.

List all the people who will be supportive of you and enlist their help. Tell all your friends that you are quitting and ask them to praise you when you aren't smoking. One of my best friends who still is trying to quit by cutting back said to me, "You haven't even noticed or commented that I hardly ever smoke around you anymore." She was right. I really hadn't noticed because I have become more used to being around people who don't smoke, rather than people who do. NOT smoking is the norm. I'm trying to be more supportive now.

This brings me to my next point (one my friend has not quite accepted): don't try to taper off; the nicotine level in your system will be just high enough to keep you in a constant state of craving and withdrawal. When you quit, quit!

Don't deceive yourself by switching to cigarettes which are low in tar and nicotine. A Stanford University Medical Center study involving 700 smokers found that people generally negated any potential health benefits by smoking more of them, inhaling more deeply, and smoking them down to a shorter butt. This, indeed, was how I worked myself up from 1 1/2 packs to two packs to three packs.

Having trouble getting yourself on the side of the fence where you want to quit even one percent more than you want to smoke?

Think about how much harder it is becoming every day to find places where smokers are welcome. A number of states—including Alaska, Connecticut, Florida, Maine, Minnesota, Montana, Nebraska, New Hampshire, New Jersey and Utah—have laws regulating smoking at private work places. Many cities in other states have tough anti-smoking ordinances. Many more are on the way. It is such a relief not to have to worry about that.

Got any children? Authorities say they metabolize secondhand tobacco smoke faster than adults. With Phil, I definitely could tell the difference in the number of colds and sore throats he got when he was living with me (after I quit) and when he was living with his father and his stepmother, both of whom smoked.

It still staggers me to read statistics attributing $23.3 billion a *year* more in direct medical costs for smokers than for non-smokers. One study stated that early smoking-related deaths cost our country $21.1 billion in earned income. What an incredible waste!

If you have a relapse and start smoking again, don't punish yourself. Be very kind and loving and start your plan all over again. Do it a third time, a fourth time, whatever is needed. Eventually, you'll find yourself in The Smoker Who is Not Currently Smoking stage, The Ex-Smoker Stage, and finally, there you'll be at The Non-Smoker Stage. A happy person with pink lungs!

COCAINE

About the Author

Charlie McMordie was such a heavy drug user that eventually suicide seemed like his only escape. He drank heavily, used marijuana, LSD, speed, and other drugs, but it was cocaine that led to his downfall. He shot, snorted, and smoked cocaine until it cost him his marriage, job, family, friends, and fortune. Although family oil and cattle brought him more than $12,000 per month for some time, most of that money was spent on drugs.

For the 15 years he was addicted, McMordie did not think he had a drug problem. The grand mal seizures, ruined relationships, and constant use were second nature to him; his entire life centered around cocaine. He reluctantly entered treatment as a result of family intervention, and he continued to deny having a drug problem until an incredible event ended his resistance.

Charlie McMordie no longer drinks or uses any drugs. He believes that so much as a single puff of marijuana could lead him back to cocaine and certain death. He now works as a counselor with chemically dependent individuals and finds true happiness and meaning helping others who are struggling in their own recoveries.

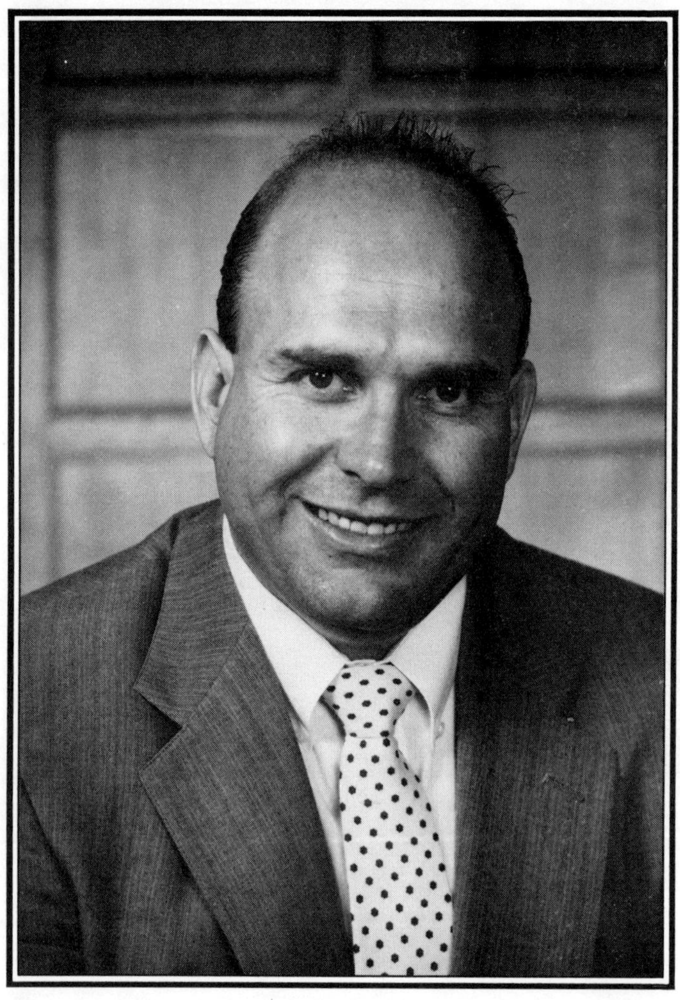

Charlie McMordie

Silhouette of a Snowman

by

Charlie McMordie with Leigh Cohn

***

Introduction

I once shot up a whole ounce of cocaine in three days. During that weekend, I probably gave myself more than one hundred injections. I started on a Friday after work—one shot after another. The insanity of addiction is to keep doing more. This was to be the time where I would be able to keep doing cocaine until I wouldn't have to do another shot. I filled the spoon completely, barely able to get any water into it. After drawing it into the syringe, I'd have this dialogue in my mind, "Isn't that too much? No, I can handle it. Shouldn't I save some for later? No, do it all now." After pushing the plunger down, before the rush took control, I remember thinking that if I died it would be over, and I'd be free. Everything went white. I fell off the commode, and had a seizure. When I woke up in the next room, not knowing how I got there, I pulled myself up and instinctively went back into the bathroom again. After nearly dying, I was standing there fixing another shot. I saw a sick person in the mirror, and I knew then that I had to change or die. The only answer seemed to be to leave the syringe alone, but not until I had finished the ounce.

From grade school until my early thirties, I habitually drank alcohol, smoked marijuana, used amphetamines, dropped hundreds of tabs of LSD, and took more varieties of pills than I can possibly remember. Cocaine was the most insidious of the lot, and my addiction to it cost me a fortune, ended my marriage, tore me away from my parents, and stripped me of any dignity I might have had. Only after quitting drugs and alcohol have I begun to experience happiness in my life.

Dual Identity

I was six when my parents were divorced, and that had a tremendous impact on me. They often fought, which always had a traumatic affect on me. When I started school, I used to tell people that my dad was dead because I was too ashamed to say that they were divorced. I lived with my mother and older brother in West, Texas, which is 70 miles south of Dallas. She didn't get alimony or child support, and she worked hard to get by.

I spent summers at my father's family ranch in Canadian, Texas, which is in the Panhandle. I stayed with my grandparents, who were pillars of the community, socially and financially well-set. They were a well-known, established ranching family with a spread of 24,000 acres of oil-filled land. There were times when my father wasn't there, but I idolized him anyway. The absence made the love stronger. I tended to overlook his shortcomings and magnify his assets. He was everything I wanted to be. I missed him deeply.

Most of my friends in West were from humble, middle class, Czechoslovakian backgrounds which was a big cultural contrast to my life in Canadian. So, as I grew up, I had two completely different backgrounds. Though confusing for me, my two identities served me in different ways. There were times in West that my head was in Canadian, and I felt elite and confident; and at other times, on the ranch, I wanted to fit in with the majority, who were not wealthy land owners like my family. In my heart, I didn't have roots or a clear identity.

I clung to the hope that my parents would remarry, that we would be a happy family, even though my father had remarried. When that dream finally died, which was around eighth grade, I started drinking. The hope of reconciliation had carried me for my early years, and once I shattered the picture of us united on the ranch, I needed something else. Booze became that replacement. I ate lunch at my grandparents' house, on my mother's side, a couple of times each week. My grandfather methodically drank one jigger of whiskey every day, never more than that one shot, and I decided to give it a try to see what would happen. I waited until I was alone, poured some into a small bottle and took it to school. My best friend and I snuck into the restroom, where I took my first drink. It tasted terrible, but it made me seem cool. Within two or three months, I was going out drinking every weekend with my friends. Alcohol gave me a connection to the popular, older crowd. By drinking, I had acceptance. From the point that I took that first drink to the day when I looked at myself and realized I was getting drunk every day was a short time.

The first time I came home drunk, I had been drinking cherry vodka, which was really disgusting—I never drank that again. I went directly to the bathroom and puked up all this red stuff, and my mother came in and asked what was the matter. I told her I got sick from a soda drinking contest, and she just accepted my answer. There were numerous times that she caught me drunk and took my lies; it was many years before she finally quit listening. She wanted to believe that I was her fair-haired child. People generally liked me. I had a charismatic personality and easily made friends because I was outgoing and personable. In a relatively short period of time, my drinking image was master of ceremonies, comedian, macho, and indestructible. I was also irresponsible, a liar and thief; and, on the inside, I was hardly the fearless leader that I seemed. Other kids in school looked at me and thought I was "cool" and particularly with my Czech friends it was somehow admirable that I drank. Most of those guys drank from an early age, so drinking made me able to fit in.

Drugs in the In-Group

I was a freshman in high school in 1967, around the time that drugs came to West. My friends and I started making trips to Dallas on weekends. I'd come home, pretend to go to sleep, and then sneak out with my buddies. There were six or seven of us who spent those years partying together. One of my friends came up with the idea of drinking cough syrup with codeine. We'd drive to one of the toughest neighborhoods in Dallas, to a pharmacy where you only had to sign your name to buy Robitussin A.C. over-the-counter. Vagrants and junkies littered the street, milling around outside of the pharmacy. It was scary and exciting at the same time. We'd drink a whole bottle of that stuff and get a little high. The biggest rush came from the act of going there, driving an hour and a half or two hours with the gang, being in this threatening environment and scoring the cough syrup, all without my mother even knowing I was out of the house. We were into these trips to Dallas and drinking cough syrup for about six months. In Dallas, we also went to all-night clubs at four and five in the morning. There'd be bands and dancers, and it was thrilling for a bunch of small town kids to be a part of this seedy underside of the big city.

Part of these social rites of passage was to court danger. For excitement, a few of us burglarized a liquor store one night while it was closed. That was a crazy, spur of the moment decision. Someone said, "Hey, let's go rob something." We'd been drinking, broke in the front door, and proceeded to load our station wagon with cases of whiskey. We also cleaned out the cash register, and we laughed hysterically when the getaway car was so filled with boxes that we couldn't get back in!

I used to hang out with all of these guys, but I did have one girl friend from eighth grade through most of college. We used to drink and do drugs together, but I was always insanely jealous of her. It was a clinging, co-dependent kind of relationship. I never wanted her to do anything without me, and if we weren't together I was afraid she was sneaking out on me with someone else. This was the first of many destructive relationships I had with women. My male friends were more important to me, and it got to be a burden hanging out with her. The rest of the guys didn't date much, so my having a girlfriend was an ego boost for me, and in some ways put me above them.

Around 1968, I began using LSD and marijuana. Actually, it was safer to have acid than weed, because marijuana was a felony while LSD was only a misdemeanor. For the next four or five years I ate acid five or six times per week. My first trip was from acid that we bought at a rock concert in Dallas. Drugs were always available at concerts. This was a small orange pill that was supposed to be split four ways. I wasn't sure that I wanted to try it, because of it's bad reputation. I'd heard that it might cause chromosome damage, so I was afraid of it. I cut the pill into pieces with my fingernail and gave everyone in the car a small piece, except I didn't take one. I just ate what was left under my fingernail. I remember thinking, "This shit doesn't do anything!" I was driving and they were all laughing and saying that they were seeing things, but I thought they were just making it all up. When I got home, I laid down on my bed and looked at an air conditioning vent on the ceiling. It started moving around and I kept staring at it. My eyes started getting a strange feeling, and beautiful colors were appearing out of the vent hole. They were distinct and unique, and I lay there enjoying it. All of a sudden, a bearded monk came to my bedside wearing a long robe. I couldn't see his face, but I thought that it was Jesus Christ visiting me. I thought that this was how people had visions. I didn't have a strongly religious background, and I was frightened at first, but that was one special experience. After that I started eating a lot of acid.

There was a cultural revolution going on. We had escape through drugs and sex whenever we wanted it. At some point most people quit playing and grew up, but I didn't. The whole time I was drinking and using I was a child in an adult's body. My mom knew I was drinking, but I kept my drug use from her. I'd always heard things about the hippies in San Francisco and the flower children, and my friends and I wanted to be that way, too, in our own hometown. In a way, drugs were a connection to the rest of our generation. We'd eat acid and walk the streets of West, banded together, without anyone knowing we were tripping. It was a great, inside joke. Thomas Wolfe's book, *The Electric Kool-Aid Acid Trip*, was popular then, and we saw ourselves as the Texas version of "the band of the merry pranksters." We patterned ourselves after that image.

When some of my friends started shooting speed, I remember thinking, "That's one thing I'll never do, I'll never get that bad." The word "never" is puzzling, and wanting to believe that "never" actually meant *NEVER* was as far as I went. As a child I was terrified of needles, and many times had to be chased around doctors' offices. But the first time I shot-up was a whole different experience, still crystal clear to me. I remember the house, the friends who were there and that it was raining. The substance was desoxin with a yellow, honey-like consistency. Someone had stolen it from a drug store. This time, I didn't run or cry; instead, I willingly offered my arm to the needle. Once again, I was doing something frightening for a thrill. I really didn't know what to expect, but I was instantly in love with shooting speed. The small prick of the needle, the blood in the syringe, the plunger down, and I was charged, alive, no task was too great. It was more exciting and the rush much stronger than eating speed had ever been. When you take speed, the central nervous system is accelerated and the heart rate increases. To me it felt like a continuous orgasm. With that exhilaration, a little part of me said, "You've crossed a line and there's no way you can ever go back." A voice also said, "There's no reason to go back, this is the answer."

Even on that first day I wanted to do more, and I took two more hits. I wanted to show everyone there that I could do more speed than they could. I did that with beer, whiskey, and acid. I not only wanted to be accepted, I wanted to be better. That attitude went back to money and the ranch. Even though I lived in this little town and worked in a store for 90 cents an hour, I knew that someday I would get the legacy and fortune from my father's family.

The more I shot speed, the more money I needed. LSD had been cheap, but crystal was expensive. We generally bought $100 bags and four or five of us would split it, but, at that time, $20 or $25 was a lot of money to me. During my junior and senior years of high school, in order to pay for the speed, we did some stealing, and I naturally slid into selling drugs. I had contacts in Fort Worth and Dallas where I would buy a pound of weed for about $90. I'd sell off most of it, keep some to smoke, and still make $70 on the pound. By then, a lot of people were getting stoned, and I was selling to friends and their friends. Weed was good to sell, too, because there would be no way of smoking a whole pound up before it got sold. With a $100 bag of speed, I would sell off half, make $50 and still have a lot for myself. But sometimes I would shoot the whole stash before I sold any. Besides providing me with money for dope, dealing also added to the image I was trying to portray. It gave me a feeling of importance and more of that instant acceptance that I thought I needed so badly.

By 1972, I had flunked out of my first college, and entered a community college near West. By that time, I was selling a couple of pounds of weed per week and had established myself as the town dealer. Whenever anyone wanted drugs, they'd come to me. My friends and I rode around a lot on country roads, drank beer, smoked dope, and listened to music. Usually, we'd eat acid late at night, talk and look at the sky, and basically just hang out together. Often, someone would get scared and then the whole group would come together to help this guy back to sanity. It was a form of male bonding. Like so many times before, one night my friends and I drove out on a dark, country road to fix some speed. The inside light of the car was on and we were trying to find veins when flashing lights from the highway patrol appeared behind us. We got busted for having controlled substances: LSD, speed, and a synthetic designer drug, MDA. We also had about a half-pound of marijuana with us, which was the only felony possession. That was the first time I'd ever gotten any cocaine, which I didn't get to try because we ditched it when the bust started.

The bust happened on Mother's Day, and it was the first time my mother learned of my drug use. When she bailed me out, I believed that I'd learned my lesson, that I'd never do it again. She accepted that response from me, and in fact I did stay pretty straight for six months of probation. Actually, I did keep getting drunk, but I stayed away from drugs and my friends. I mainly spent time with my girlfriend, in that same volatile relationship. We'd fight and make up, fight and make up, mainly because of my jealousy.

Cocaine and Family Money

Compared to alcohol, cough syrup with codeine, marijuana, LSD, speed, and other pills, cocaine fit in right at the top. The hallucinogenic drugs that I had been doing started to scare me. I wasn't able to maintain the mental control needed to stay detached from the drug experiences and had too many bad trips. My irrational thinking built up until I'd think I would never be able to regain my senses and that I'd keep hallucinating for the rest of my life. That terrified me! I thought I'd have to be institutionalized and would be certified as "crazy."

Cocaine started as a small part of my poly-drug use. Being from humble means in West, cocaine seemed wasteful because it was more expensive than the other drugs and it didn't last as long. During my final years of college, cocaine started taking hold of me. I bought it to sell, but I'd never make any money from it. If I didn't immediately get rid of the whole stash, I'd use it all. I had no control over it from the very beginning. From those early days on, I shot it, too, and rarely snorted it except in social situations. Also, unlike my other drug experiences, most of the time I used cocaine by myself. I always set myself up to do it the way I wanted to do it. At college, the group I hung out with weren't into needles, and I didn't really want them to know how much I was shooting up. In those early years, I used as much cocaine as I could get. I would shoot a gram in a couple of hours, which broke down to about ten shots.

My cocaine use started to accelerate during my last year of college. I broke up with my girlfriend, and I also got more involved with bigger dealers. One of the roommates in a house I lived in paid his rent with cocaine, and he became one of my main drug connections. I flaunted my cocaine involvement and even had a baseball cap with the word "Snow" embroidered on it. I was infatuated with the drug for nine years.

I started having grand mal seizures, which continued for as long as I kept doing drugs. A grand mal seizure is like an epileptic attack: convulsions, a total tensing of the body, and usually I'd pass out from the stress on my nervous system. Sometimes I had them in public, which embarrassed me terribly, especially in front of my friends.

I still went to my dad's ranch during summers, and looked forward to those times because I'd get clean. Although I'd take along about a pound of weed to smoke, I wouldn't do coke, speed, or other heavy drugs while on the ranch. My brother and I drank a lot of beer up there, but compared to my normal routine I was much cleaner. I did physical labor on the ranch, learned about the business, and began to make a transition into that blue blood hierarchy.

When I graduated from college, I visited my dad in Mexico, where he was in a rest home fighting multiple sclerosis. He was also recovering from addiction using hypnosis in his cure. We talked and I thought it was good for him to be recovering, yet I did not mention my own drug abuse. Here I had tried every drug I could find for the past ten years, shot up cocaine whenever I could get my hands on it, and I didn't think I had a problem!

We also talked about my future, and paved my way into the family business. A soft, high paying job with the power and prestige of working as an heir in an old ranching family seemed to assure me of success. Actually, the reality of the job was not what I expected. The long lunches, high rise offices with secretaries, and meetings with bankers turned out to be taking orders from my uncle, cleaning soured feed out of cattle feeders, putting out hay, and giving shots to calves. I'd seen other guys move in to their family businesses, and they'd be flying private airplanes and riding in expensive cars. I always expected that I would do the same thing. Instead, I was paid $450 per month, got a small house, free meat, and a used pickup truck.

I worked with my family for close to three years and, surprisingly, enjoyed starting at the ground floor. I felt at home with the middle class workers because these were the kinds of people I grew up with in West, and they respected me for working there.

While I was still in college the most cocaine I'd buy would be a half-ounce, which cost about $1000. I'd put aside half of that, uncut, for myself; then I'd cut the rest with lactose for my friends. But when I moved to the ranch in 1977, I had more money to spend. After about a year, I got more involved with the business and started making commissions. It wasn't unusual for me to take home $6000 per month in bonuses. I'd buy an ounce of cocaine at a time for personal use, or I'd share it with one friend who lived nearby. He would snort and I'd shoot. We used to fly in his private plane to Oklahoma City in the middle of the night to score coke. While he was flying, I'd be snorting and making rails for him. Once again, I was flirting with danger, except the stakes kept getting higher. Besides the obvious risks, if we got caught my whole relationship with my father's family and the money would have gotten blown.

Money and the power it brings is another addiction which took control. It provided me with the same things dope did: arrogance, a grandiose self-esteem, and the idea that nothing was too much or too good for me. Besides my pay, I was drawing about $3000 per month from a trust fund, and they were drilling more and more gas and oil wells on the property. For a while in the early 1980s I was getting up to $12,000 per month from my share just for breathing! A lot of the money went into my arm. I bought ounces of cocaine every few weeks. It was during this period that I shot that ounce in three days.

After I finally broke up with my girlfriend of so many years, I dated several women but did not have any serious relationships. Then I met a wonderfully happy young woman while I was working in Canadian. She came from another ranching family, that also had oil and money. We seemed destined to get together—nobility marrying nobility. She never used drugs, and the most she ever drank was an occasional beer or glass of wine. She represented to me a chance for happiness.

Marriage Versus Cocaine

I saw problems with my cocaine abuse, and even before we married I had slowed down a little so that I stopped shooting and snorted less. My uncle, who ran the business, moved me to a huge ranch in the middle of nowhere. When I got the chance, I'd go to Amarillo and party with lawyers, bankers, and rich professionals who I'd met through business. The cocaine flowed in those circles, but they all snorted it, and so I did, too. That was okay. I wasn't using heavily, and I fit in well socially. My future wife knew I did some coke, but she didn't know the whole story. She didn't understand why I used, but she didn't condemn me for it either.

Before we had married, I had a talk with her father who asked me about my cocaine use. I'm not sure how the subject came up. I assured him that cocaine was a thing of the past for me, that I was completely off drugs. One of the reasons that marrying her appealed to me was that, in the back of my mind, I knew that if I screwed up with my family, I could always fall back on her family's money for my future. At the time this was not a conscious realization, but looking back I know that this was something that I considered.

Living away on that ranch made me isolated and lonely. After six or eight months of dating, we decided to get married. I was five days late for our wedding. Some friends came up from Amarillo and decided we should celebrate. They brought a couple of women with them, and we went nude sunbathing, roped steers, smoked dope, and stayed drunk. My soon-to-be wife called everyday asking, "Are we going to get married today?" I'd always make up some kind of excuse. I spent a lot of time contemplating how I would explain my sunburned ass! That marriage was destined to fail. She accepted my lies and stories in much the same way my mother had when I was younger.

I eventually got fired by my uncle when I ran off to Amarillo to party. I got too messed up on coke to supervise ten truckloads of cattle that arrived. It was a major mistake, not the first one either, and it cost me my job. I felt that it was totally unfair of my uncle to fire me and placed the blame on him, refusing to take any responsibility. Newly married and angry, I decided to build my own feed lot and go into competition.

My wife and I bought a house in Canadian. I cut my drug use way back, because I knew it was a problem for me, and I was trying to make our marriage work. We had a good time while we were married, had enough money to travel, and were basically a happy couple. Our biggest problem was that I would go to bars late into the night without her. When she would call to find me, I didn't want to look weak in front of my friends, so I played defiant, macho games.

I had told her that I wouldn't do any more coke. But after we had been married for a little while, I asked a friend of mine to send me an ounce of coke, which he did, wrapped in a shirt. I showed the shirt to my wife, knowing that the coke was hidden inside. I split the ounce in half, hid one package away, and couldn't wait for the chance to be alone with it. When she was ready for bed, I said I was going to stay up for awhile to watch television. She believed me. I snorted as much as I could and had another grand mal seizure. The next thing I remember was waking up, the family doctor giving me a shot of Valium and Demerol to slow down my heart rate, and my mother-in-law standing over me shaking the bag of dope in my face, screaming, "Is this all of it? Is this all of it?" I was busted! The very next day, the whole scene played again: my secret using with the second bag, the grand mal seizure, mother-in-law, doctor, everything.

The day after that, they took me to Denver for treatment. I went with a bad attitude and cynically took tests and talked to psychiatrists. I knew I had a problem with cocaine—the grand mal seizures convinced me of that. However, I didn't think I had any problem with weed or booze, and I saw no connection between my addiction to cocaine and my poly-drug usage. They recommended treatment for me at that time, but I decided not to enter a facility or start therapy. I believed I could stop using on my own. I thought I had enough willpower to do anything, and my wife and her family, who knew nothing about addiction, believed me.

We returned home to Canadian, this time to a more strained marriage. The news was out, and, in such a small town, there were a lot of questions from family and others. I kept to my claim that I knew I had a problem but could get over it alone, and everyone was happy to hear that I was trying to stay straight.

I continued going to bars and smoked grass, which kept me in "bad company." One day, a friend's uncle was drunk and started a fight with my friend, who shot and killed him. I was the only eyewitness. The trauma of that night made it unbearable to even watch violence on television anymore. It upset me more than I could have expected. Again, word travels fast in small towns, and the rumors included tales of dope deals and drug addiction. My friend was charged with first degree murder, and I helped him get a lawyer to defend him. After many postponements, the case finally came to trial. Before I testified, the District Attorney took me to the back of the courtroom and intimidated me about telling the truth. There had been more rumors, this time about my supposedly bribing the judge, and he shook me up. When it came time for me to testify on my friend's behalf, I claimed I couldn't remember what had happened, and basically choked in my testimony. That night, I told my friend's lawyer about what the D.A. had done to shake me up, and the next day I told the whole truth about the shooting and the D.A.'s coercion. My friend was exonerated.

I couldn't take the pressure of the trial, went back to my banker and lawyer friends, and started snorting cocaine again. My dream of opening a feed lot failed to materialize. It got built, but never saw any cattle. I wasn't working anywhere, and went back and forth to Amarillo for cocaine. When I started using again, the pain was too great for my wife. Although she truly did love me, she walked out. She didn't want to see me on the floor again, and she wouldn't wait around for me to die.

Living on the Edge

For the next few years, I lived off of my trust without really working much. I stayed loaded most of the time. Life became one continuous party. One time I went to Tampa and Jamaica with a girlfriend and spent $10,000 in two weeks, mainly on drugs. I went broke three or four times, hocked jewelry and cameras, and had money wired to me by my bank in Canadian. That was the only time I freebased cocaine. Freebasing is like a furnace that burns money. The process uses more cocaine than any other method, and it's gone quicker. I didn't like freebasing much, but kept doing it for the two weeks we were on that trip. I hated seeing so much coke wasted by freebasing. It took about a quarter of an ounce just to start cooking, but the rush was a lot like shooting up. I became so pathetic there that I tried to hock my diamond ring, a family heirloom worth $15,000, for an ounce of cocaine, but the Rastafarian wasn't interested in getting yet another tourist's ring. When we got back to Florida, I had 36 cents in my pocket and a hot credit card. I dropped that girl off in Amarillo, went to Dallas, picked up another date, went to a Rolling Stones concert, and continued partying.

A while later, I went back to Amarillo to see my girlfriend there. We tried to check into a motel that I usually stayed at, but the clerk wouldn't rent me a room. He later claimed that I grabbed him by his tie, pulled him across the counter, and hit him in the face. I didn't remember any of that, although I do recall pushing his cash register to the floor. A little while later, I was arrested for felony destruction of private property. It cost me $7000 to get out of that jam.

In 1982, I moved to Dallas and did nothing but get drunk, snort coke, and deal drugs. I snorted about half of an ounce per week, selling off the remainder. I'd occasionally skip a day or two to rest, but otherwise would stay wired all day and night for days on end. My greatest fears then were of dying or going to jail, yet everything I did pushed me in those directions. As always, I lived dangerously close to the edge.

The beginning of the end came that December. My trust, which was bringing me $8000-10,000 per month, paid a bonus of $40,000. I started into a four-month party for myself and everybody around me. I started shooting cocaine again, spent New Year's Eve taking a large group of friends to a $100 per seat party where whiskey and flake flowed, and kept going at that pace. Five days later, I scored quaaludes at a Dallas bar, knowing that they would help me get some well-needed sleep. After more drinking and pills, I left the bar and drove into a tree. After regaining consciousness, I called a cab from a convenience store, and ended up in a fist fight with the driver before he took me home. The Dallas police arrived shortly thereafter. Another arrest for unlawful possession, confiscation of the $5000 cash from my billfold, more lawyers and money spent, and I was off and running again. By February, 1983, my bank account was $15,000 overdrawn, but I kept using and spending.

Finally, I couldn't even shoot enough dope to stay awake and took 150 milligrams of valium in my apartment with a strung out, 19 year old woman I'd been seeing for a few weeks. We slept soundly. I awoke at seven in the morning to a phone call from my dad. He and my stepmother were concerned about me. They had heard from the bank about my spending, had tried to reach me for days, and called early in hope of finding me. I tried to sound happy and together, but as I looked out of my bedroom window, I noticed that the apartment complex was on fire. I was in shock and said to him, "This son-of-a-bitch is on fire!" He responded by asking what drugs I had taken, but this was no hallucination! I woke the girl, grabbed a few belongings and my stash, and simply walked out of the building. I went across the street, shot up some more coke, got a couple of six-packs of beer and left. I took her home, paranoid that she might have started the fire, and continued to get loaded. If my dad had not called, I doubt if I would have awakened.

That day I checked in and out of five different hotels. Everywhere I went, I smelled smoke. It seemed to keep following me. In each place I shot up, but kept moving because I feared that narcotics agents or fire inspectors were out to get me busted or blame me for the fire. I couldn't sleep because I knew they'd catch up to me.

HELP!

I stopped using because the drugs only increased my crazed state. For five days I'd been off coke, I'd even thrown my weed away, but I still had not slept. I experienced hallucinations that affected my sight, smell, and hearing. I went to the airport and bought tickets to two different places for planes leaving at the same time. For no specific reason, I flew to my dad's. I got to his house at 2:00 in the morning with no clothes, no suitcase, nothing.

Before then, I had always been careful to hide my addiction from my father. I protected our relationship, showing only the charismatic, successful side of my personality. I always feared that if I blew that relationship, I'd be blowing away any chance at the big money. Because of my parents' divorce and my not seeing him much, my connection to him had more to do with money than blood. Yet, some deeper sense of security and comfort brought me to his home. For the first two or three days, I wouldn't sleep. I thought my stepmother wanted to poison me, so I only ate food that I cooked for myself. I thought I heard my dealer and father talking behind closed doors. I was beat, I'd reached the end of the line. The only viable solution for me seemed to be suicide.

Killing myself felt like the perfect answer. Everything that I saw, did, or heard confirmed that suicide offered me the best option. A certain peace came over me as I walked into my dad's bedroom. I calmly asked to use his gun to shoot myself. My stepmother, a registered nurse, knew exactly what to do. She ordered me to take a shower and put on clean clothes, and they took me to the hospital. I thought they were taking me for a legal suicide, so I wrote my last will and testament on the way. When we arrived at the hospital, I started having another grand mal seizure, right in my father's arms. He thought I was dying, and I wished that I could; but, when I came to, I knew I wanted to live.

In the emergency ward of this Amarillo psychiatric hospital, I realized how much I wanted to live. I didn't care if I had to stay in an institution forever; it didn't matter, as long as I could live. In the admitting room, the woman behind the desk asked, "What's a fine young man like yourself doing trying to get into this place?" I had no answer. I had run out of things and people to blame, and I stood silently dumbfounded. I turned to my dad and he replied to her, "Because he's a drug addict and an alcoholic." In that short, direct statement, I finally realized how screwed up I had gotten my life. It made perfect sense to me, and was my turning point.

In the hospital, they gave me drugs to control my psychotic state, the delusions and paranoia. I stayed in isolation for the first week, sedated so I could sleep and finally rest. After three weeks, I was eating and sleeping a lot better, and my thinking started to improve. My first visitors were a couple of women I'd occasionally gotten loaded with in school. When I heard that they'd been sober for over a year, I didn't believe them. They asked if I wanted to go with them to a meeting, and the excitement of getting out of the hospital even for a few hours propelled me to accept the offer. Once I got there, though, I feared that everyone knew I was a mental patient or thought I was crazy. When it came time to introduce myself to the rest of the gathering, I said, "My name is Charlie, I'm an alcoholic." I went along like that, feeling the need to fit in, but not really sure that I belonged there. Still, listening to the others substantiated that my feelings and experiences were shared by many others, and I returned regularly. The meetings showed me that people could be interested in me and care about my welfare. It was refreshing and new to hang around people who didn't want my dope or money. For my five weeks in the hospital I stayed completely clean, going to meetings, but still clinging to denial about the seriousness of my addiction.

Recovery

My doctors and family decided that I should go to a special treatment facility in San Diego. On May 18, 1983, my uncle took me to the airport, reassuring me that everything was going to be all right. About halfway to San Diego, I suddenly figured out why I had to go away, realizing, "They're sending me out there to keep me from getting drunk and loaded." Amazing! Instantly, I resisted once again and thought these exact words, "It'll be a cold day in Hell when I don't drink and get loaded." Spiritual experiences are hard to explain, but I believe that God sent me a message that day. The plane landed for a stopover in Denver, and there were two feet of snow on the ground. It may not have meant anything to the other passengers, but that snow changed my life. I saw it as God's answer that it was a cold day in Hell, today! I finally admitted to myself that I was a sick junkie who could find a greater power to help me, that I could stop using drugs and alcohol. For the rest of the flight to San Diego, I felt transformed. The internal chaos, my fears, and my paranoia were replaced by calm. I relaxed and completely believed what my uncle had said. Everything would be all right. In those few hours, my level of understanding had totally changed.

I stayed in primary detoxification for my first seventeen days in San Diego, even after going five weeks without drugs or alcohol. In the fellowship of recovery, I started seeing people who were happy. In the early meetings, I totally respected the ones who got "chips" for staying clean for thirty days. Voluntary abstinence seemed incomprehensible to me, but I wanted to stay clean, too. I stayed in the hospital for forty-five days, which made my first chip a little easier, but as I got more time under my belt—sixty, ninety days—I became more and more committed. In one sense, I was lucky. I did not crave more drugs or alcohol. I had burned out, I'd done enough.

The first step of the program was to look chronologically at my condition, its progression, unmanageablity, and my powerlessness over the disease of addiction. I had to admit total defeat. When you're using, you don't see that you're losing every time. You don't acknowledge all the harm you're doing—you can't and still continue to use. It's a tactic to look back and think, "It wasn't that bad," or "I didn't get in that much trouble," or to blame someone else. When you're using, you get by thinking that way, you protect and nurture the disease; but when you're sober you have to see just how bad it all is. When I really looked at the way my life had been going, it was devastating. I wanted to beat myself up about it. I thought, "Charlie, how could you be so stupid? Couldn't you see: four DWIs, two drug busts, ..."

I also learned that I wasn't alone anymore and never had to be again. I met and talked to people who had done even more dope than I and those who had done less. The ego-game of who could do the most no longer mattered, nor did my material possessions. The fellowship of recovery—true caring, common love for others—those are the things that mattered. Addiction brings a kind of self-centeredness that only causes pain. I found that people could be happy, joyous, and free. I envied them and aspired to be like that.

Seeing people who had been every bit as sick as I had been, and hearing them talk about their months and even years of continuous sobriety had a tremendous impact on me. I heard stories about people losing families, wives, husbands, and friends. Yet, those same people had hope, which is what I desperately needed. I had to become open to the idea that what they were all saying was true. I could find no reason for them to be lying—there would be nothing to gain—and, by telling the truth, they became comfortable and safe within the group. In the programs of recovery, I found acceptance from others. That was something I had always strived for, and the fellowship of recovery is what I had really needed during all of those years of hanging out with groups of friends. Interestingly, the same kinds of people I got loaded with became the ones I stayed sober with in recovery; now, we were helping each other instead of killing each other.

The first test of my sobriety came upon discharge from the hospital. With a little skepticism, I entered a halfway house suggested by the treatment team. The one I picked had no structure. I could sleep as late as I wanted, and I could come and go without rules. I also participated in group meetings at the hospital five days each week, which meant taking a two hour public bus ride each way. I had a tough time during that stage of my recovery, especially because I felt homesick for Texas. I spent a lot of my energy building faith in a power greater than myself and in developing the belief that everything would work out as long as I stayed away from drugs. With the passing of time, my emotions rose and dropped, but I continued on the course of sobriety. By staying in action, the process of my recovery started giving me some comfort. Instead of feeling imprisoned in California, I began to perceive its advantages.

Receiving my six-month chip proved to me that not only could I live without dope, but I could enjoy life, too. I began losing my fears of the future and started letting go of my past. As my confidence grew, the treatment team reevaluated my progress and reached the decision that I should return to Texas. This was to be my major test. The fear of transition got replaced by excitement about starting a new support group. I moved in with my mother and her husband, who also had first-hand understanding about recovery. Her involvement in my recovery led the way to our rebuilding a relationship that had deteriorated from years of my lies and drug use. I also found a job, for the first in four years, which brought me a greater sense of self-worth and responsibility.

Being clean and sober is first and foremost in my life, and only by being that way can I feel a part of a grander scheme. I continue to go to regular meetings of addicts and alcoholics. I've also made the career choice to counsel chemically-dependent individuals. But it's important to me to keep my professional life and my personal recovery separate; what I do for a living cannot be what I do to stay alive. If someone offered me cocaine now, I wouldn't give it a thought, not even a consideration. I firmly believe that if I ever used cocaine again, I'd die. Alcohol or weed are not alternatives either, because I know that with one drink or just a hit on a joint, cocaine is right around the corner ready to pounce. I've done all the using I want to do.

I don't even have relationships with people who do drugs and don't want to quit. Users are not supporters. When I was originally hospitalized in Amarillo, I had fantasies of bus loads of friends coming to visit me. Other than the women who took me to the meetings and my parents, I only had one other visitor—someone reminding me that I owed him money. I don't have much contact with my old friends, anymore. We're in different places now because most of them are still using drugs.

There's no growth or meaning when you have a tube in your nose or needle in your arm. Cocaine prevents you from living. What I get out of being straight is sharing myself openly and honestly without expectation. Trying to help others is important to me, and that just doesn't happen while using drugs. Now I have meaning in my life and it's better than it ever was before. At last, everything fits.

NARCOTICS ADDICTION

About the Author

Bob MacFarlane became addicted to injected opiates during his residency as a physician. He was expelled from his neurosurgical residency, suspended from the practice of medicine, and started and lost numerous jobs. Infections in one arm almost resulted in amputation and caused permanent damage.

During his ten years of taking narcotics, MacFarlane denied his addiction. He believed that he could stop or limit his drug use, but despite entering treatment and attempting to quit on his own, he kept returning to the needle. A miracle saved him from a deliberate, lethal overdose, but even that was not enough to stop him from continued using. After a preliminary investigation into his inordinate number of prescriptions for Talwin, he entered a chemical dependency program and started his recovery.

Bob MacFarlane has been drug-free for more than six years, during which time he has returned to medical practice and has gained notoriety as a physician in the field of chemical dependency. He is a certified "addictionologist" and has been a consultant to the Drug Enforcement Administration, the Physicians Diversion Program, and various other educational and treatment groups. Through addiction and recovery, he has found a new direction and new purpose in his life.

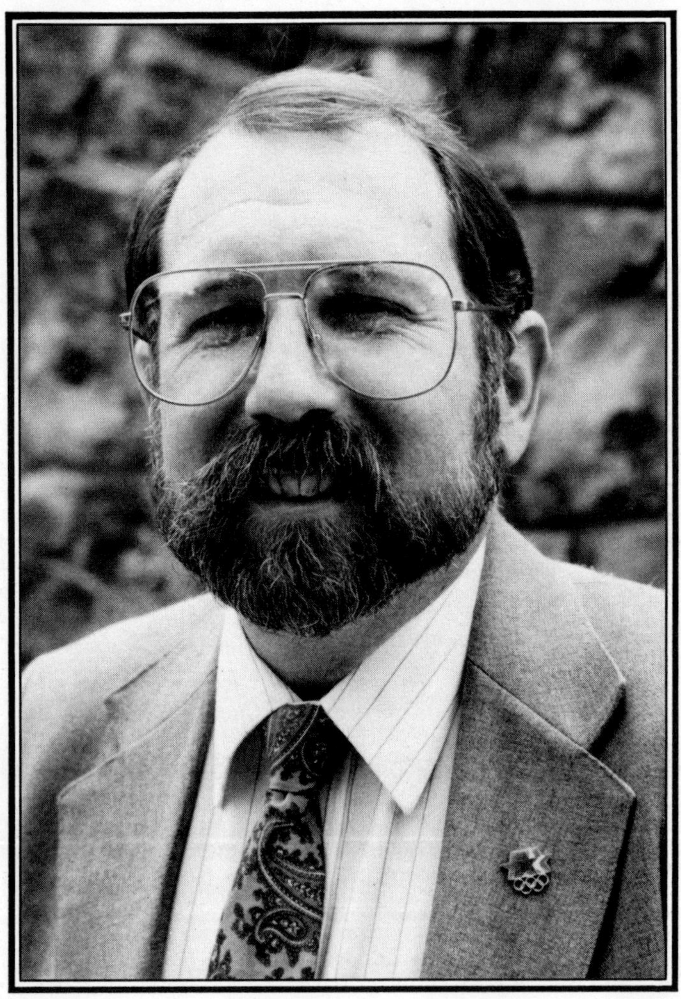

Bob MacFarlane, M.D.

Bad Medicine

by

Bob MacFarlane, M.D.

***

It Couldn't Happen to Me

I was devastated. At twenty-six years of age, I knew I could not survive the end of the year. The shock of the realization that I was a drug addict was overwhelming—too much to bear—so I began practicing what I had become adept at over the previous few months: I fell back into denial, a course which I would take in varying degrees for the next ten years of my life. In medical school I had heard of denial—a psychological defense mechanism to protect our egos from the trauma of stark reality. A mechanism normally employed in times of great stress, it is also capable of being abused and distorted to the point of allowing us to sever our connection with reality to the point of living in a fantasy world created in the bowels of our own minds. My fantasy was that I could not be a drug addict, despite objective evidence to the contrary, because I was of a superior mental and psychological fabric and thus immune to the effects of drugs which had taken many, better than I, to institutions and graves.

I, like many, had had a mental picture engraved of what a drug addict was: a spineless, weak-willed creature of dubious moral values, the product of an impoverished environment, generally from a broken home and another ethnic group, who knew nothing of the world outside his personal ghetto, and cared for nothing save his own personal comfort and pleasures. I knew that I did not fit the stereotype and therefore assumed that I was immune to the addictive properties of drugs that held lesser people in their clutches.

I was a fortunate child and had been born into and brought up in the best of households in post-war Southern California. My parents were hardworking and loving, steeped in the Protestant work ethic. They had been raised in the Great Depression without the opportunity for advanced education, but had absorbed the moral values and ethics of the times. My mother devoted herself to raising us three children while my father worked as a paint store manager six days a week. The home was an environment of love and encouragement. I was instilled with traditional moral values, involved in church and the Boy Scouts, rewarded for good behavior and punished for bad. Material things were not rained upon us, but values and opportunities were freely given. I don't mean to paint an overly rosy picture of my childhood—we were certainly not "the Waltons"—but I was spared many of the childhood traumas of those who have grown up in more dysfunctional households. I never witnessed alcoholism in the home, mental illness, child abuse or neglect, incest or any of the more devastating traumas of growing up in such an environment. We shared middle class values, lived on the "right side" of the tracks, had an intact family, and always had food on the table and a roof over our heads. I have no one to blame for the seeming tragedy to come—not my family or society, which had never wronged me. My problems were, for the most part, of my own making.

As a child, I felt special and unique and somehow different from other children my age. I frequently pondered my uniqueness and why I was here. I came to the conclusion that I was a special emissary. Whether from Heaven or Hell, I knew not which, but I knew I had some special mission in life. At times I was noble of spirit; at others, I acted out in antisocial ways. I seemed to enjoy being bad on occasion, and revelled in violating the rules if I thought I could get away with it (nothing more serious than the proverbial pigtails in the inkwell, mind you). After all, since I was special, why should I be bound by the rules that govern other mortals?

At eight years of age, I decided to become a doctor and felt I had discovered my *raison d'être*. I felt a sense of purpose and direction in my life at that point and never waivered from my ambition. Being driven by a single-minded purpose, I became obsessed with reaching my goal. That obsession (magnificent or mundane), I believe now, prevented me from falling prey to my drug addiction at a much earlier age.

I was exposed to a variety of drugs from childhood on and, although not developing an identifiable dependency at that time, I now realize that I reacted differently even then. The patent "snake bite medicine" I was given when I had the measles had a definite, memorable effect on me. My physical discomforts were quickly forgotten and supplanted by a wonderful sense of well-being and euphoria. Likewise, the solvents in my high school chemistry lab stockroom (and at home in our garage), my first drinking experience in high school, experimentation with marijuana in college, use of diet pills to help me study, and unsupervised trials of anaesthetics in medical school: each experience was a red-letter day in my life. Intoxication, in and of itself, was an experience of spiritual magnitude to be sought after as a pleasurable alternative to the more mundane vagaries of life. I loved it, yet I denied myself its seduction as my obsession to achieve far outweighed my desire to wallow in the hedonistic luxuries of chemical wantonness.

In college during the sixties I looked upon my peers who used drugs with disdain. I self-righteously felt superior to those who I felt must use drugs to enjoy life. I set myself up as a self-denying ascetic for the sake of achieving my monomaniacal goal, telling myself I must sacrifice the pleasures of the flesh for better, more ethereal things.

This approach to my studies paid dividends in that I excelled academically. Doing well in college, I attended the medical school of my choice on a scholarship, graduating in the top of my class, and was president of the honor society. My future seemed assured. I had gained the respect and admiration of my peers and they perceived me as "down on drugs." Many of them voiced surprise when they later found out about my addiction; I seemed the least likely candidate to go down that road.

My ascetic lifestyle had other, unsought results: I became less socially active and more and more reclusive, which helped to set me up for my descent when my life fell precipitously apart. When I had achieved my great and noble goal, and had graduated in 1971 with my new title of "Doctor," I made a startling and devastating discovery: I didn't like medicine!

Into the Abyss

As an intern in a prestigious West Coast hospital, I began to realize that my chosen career in the field of medicine was not what I had expected. I had entered medical training as a naive young idealist, hoping somehow to play an important role as a healer and help relieve the suffering of the world. In hindsight, it was more likely that I chose the medical profession to overcome my own feelings of inadequacy through reverence by my fellow man as a great healer, rather than any noble, selfless desire to alleviate suffering.

I did not witness the noble virtues in my colleagues.Unlike the Dr. Kildares of the screen, rather they were overworked, cynical technicians seemingly more obsessed with academicism and peer-approval than patient care. While deriding the apparent faults of my colleagues, I was becoming exactly what I saw in them. I was becoming cold and insensitive to the needs of others. My values deteriorated and I began perceiving patients as an intrusion on my time and a burden to my serenity. I became more self-centered and sought out the baser pleasures of life. The practice of medicine lost its attraction. I had not received the recognition and respect I had felt I earned, and instead was treated (as interns are) with some degree of contempt by those placed more favorably in the medical hierarchy. Even my patients rarely treated me with the respect and dignity I thought I deserved.

My disillusionment with medicine escalated, and so did my moral degeneration. I thought nothing of self-medicating minor ailments I imagined I might have. I paid little attention to the adage that the physician who treats himself has a fool for a patient. Pills were freely available to us in medical training at that time, and I took what was available. I did not perceive any pattern in my use and never would think of using while on duty, which allowed me to persist in the delusion that I couldn't have a problem.

Perhaps it was inevitable that, believing myself immune, I would seek out better and more efficacious drugs. And so it was. One evening, while on the urology service, I gave an unfortunate young man with a kidney stone a few milligrams of morphine intravenously. Formerly moaning and writhing in great pain, he suddenly relaxed and a calm smile came over his face. My curiosity was piqued. I had known the pharmacological effects of morphine as a pain killer, but this demonstration was phenomenal. I took the remainder of the ampule home that night and, when off duty, took it myself. Its action on me was likewise phenomenal; suddenly everything in my life that appeared somewhat out of place became understandable, tolerable and uniform. I seemed to be able to soar above the tiresome banalities of my life. The vicissitudes of my existence were overcome. The universe took on new meaning and the harmony of the spheres became apparent. I experienced something seemingly sacred and holy that only the few which have known the drug's seduction can comprehend. I thought I had found the answer, yet morally I knew I could not repeat the experience without suffering the mental turmoil one must when violating personal ethics.

Nevertheless, a week or so later, I found an opportunity, again off duty, to repeat the experience with Demerol, another narcotic. Easily justified, having convinced myself that this was only an experiment to compare the effects of two commonly prescribed pain medications, I carried out the act with alacrity and obtained similar results. The physical differences were minimal, and I carefully noted them, but the spiritual experience was identical. Again I had found that place from whence I did not want to return, like Coleridge with his Xanadu. And like Coleridge I had sealed my fate with the curse of Morpheus.

Over the next few months, my "experiments" became more frequent—each time I had a night off I returned to the dominion of the needle. After trying all the narcotics available, I settled with Talwin, a narcotic believed to be "nonaddicting" then and therefore available without restriction in the hospital. It became my drug of choice primarily because it was not a controlled substance at that time and no one bothered to keep track of it. When supplies ran low, it was simply reordered, and no one seemed to take note of its rapid disappearance.

Within three months, I found myself using it in the mornings prior to going on duty. I had ever-increasing periods of anxiety, stomach pains and chills which only seemed to be relieved by more Talwin. I was slipping more rapidly into the abyss of addiction but could not accept the facts. I blamed my frequent abstinence symptoms on recurrent bouts of the "flu." I took to wearing long sleeve shirts to cover the needle marks and bruises, primarily so I wouldn't have to see them and be faced with what I really had become. I found myself becoming less responsible at work, living a lie in my attempt to appear normally functional, but disappearing at odd times to inject myself. I made excuses for over-utilization of restrooms, swelling of the hands, excessive tardiness, unpredictable moodiness, and deterioration of personal hygiene and appearance. But the lies I told others did not compare with the lies I told myself.

Self-deceit becomes an art form in addicts and I was a prodigy in that arena. I convinced myself I could "control it," I was not addicted and was just temporarily medicating some as yet undiagnosed stress disorder. I knew I was just tired and over-stressed, as are all interns, working shifts of thirty-six hours on and twelve off. I thought my symptoms were the cause of my self-medication and not the result, as I was later to find.

Finally, the reality of my situation became apparent. I could no longer deny my addiction when I was using in the morning to get going, at night to go to sleep, and throughout the day as the need seemed to arise. My awareness vacillated, and in brief periods of clarity, I became shocked by the fact that I was practicing medicine while under the influence of drugs: assisting at surgery, performing invasive procedures, intervening in life-threatening situations, ordering potent medications, diagnosing illnesses, and being awakened and giving orders over the phone in a drug-induced stupor. The realization frightened me that I had the power of life and death, the power to heal or maim, and was forfeiting it because the drug had become more important than anything else in my life. My obsession with it replaced all my normal drives, interests and concerns. My only real care was obtaining more, insuring my supply, and using as much as I dared without being caught or causing someone else great harm.

The realization that I was indeed addicted (but not an "addict," mind you), forced me to take action. Enjoying the drug with the passion I did was inconsistent with my own moral code and my desire to pursue a self-sacrificing career in medicine. I made multiple attempts to stop on my own but failed miserably on each occasion. I only dared take off from work two days at a time which was never enough time to return to any semblance of normalcy, and I feared a longer leave would arouse suspicion. These vain attempts were marked by abdominal pain and cramping, joint pains, shaky chills, and violent jerks that would awake me from the little sleep I got. The worst part, however, seemed to be the overwhelming anxiety and fears associated with the withdrawal. As the time approached to return to work, my fears would obtain mastery of my soul and I would panic at the thought of working in such a state. The only tenable plan to my deluded mind, would be to return to the use of Talwin, untill my next opportunity to quit. By this time I was nearing the end of my internship and had a one week break coming, so I tried to hold out untill then.

I had secured a residency in neurosurgery and hoped the change would be conducive to getting away from drugs. During my one week hiatus, I moved from Torrance to San Diego and managed to quit using for a few days prior to starting my new position. I was still in withdrawal then and found I had to use from time to time to get by. In no time at all, I was back to my old pattern of frequent daily use.

One of my first trials by fire was scrubbing on three craniotomies in one night. I found with the length of the cases, I was going into withdrawal before the end of each. The first symptoms were running eyes and nose followed by fits of sneezing. The paper masks we used didn't hold up well with repeated sneezing. This and other minor irritations, coupled with my awareness that I couldn't seem to stop or control my use on my own, drove me to seek treatment for the first time. I had only been using intravenous narcotics for a few months by this time, but the tombstones had already appeared in my eyes and I felt hopelessly lost.

I sought the counsel of a psychiatry resident who I felt I could trust, who initially reacted in an unsettling manner, seeming very uncomfortable with the situation. He later was a suicide victim, and I wonder if he had been chemically dependent at the time and thus threatened. He referred me to a private psychiatrist in the community, who was very respected and tried his best, but neither he nor I had an inkling of what we were up against. He placed me in a locked psychiatric facility for several days, at which time I informed him I was adequately detoxified and felt I would never return to the use of drugs. I fully believed this to be the truth at the time and he appeared to agree. I merrily returned home with a new lease on life and nary a thought of using drugs until I came upon a few "empty" vials. I immediately became overwhelmed with a compulsion to gather, drop by drop, the residual from each and amass enough to use. I was right back to where I had left off.

Of Derelicts and Tapeworms

I made multiple other attempts to stop over the next year and a half, each time generally less successful than the last. I took as much time off as I dared and at other times tried to stop while I continued to work. The latter method inevitably ended in disaster. I would find myself invariably in an emergent situation at the height of my withdrawal and would frequently flee from the situation to seek out more drugs. After swearing off "forever," each relapse became a greater defeat and I felt more and more helpless. The veil of denial was occasionally pierced with the realization that I could not do it on my own, which just added more anxiety to my desperation, since I did not dare jeopardize my career by turning myself in for treatment again.

The very thing I feared was realized when, unable to hide my addiction any longer, I was discovered leaving paraphernalia about hospital restrooms and confronted by the Chief of Neurosurgery. I was relieved of my duties as a second year resident and referred for psychiatric treatment again. This time I was placed in a psychiatric unit for thirty days. Initially elated at the opportunity, I returned to using on the unit following my first pass outside. Caught, I sheepishly refused transfer to a more highly structured, locked unit and, having failed treatment, was not invited back to my training program. Up to that point, I had performed over one hundred neurosurgical procedures and assisted on many more while under the influence of drugs and persisted in the delusion that as soon as I got things together they would knock down my door to invite me back!

I spent the next year foundering about, not working, and taking advantage of my friends—people who had believed in me and tried very hard to assist me in my recovery. In each case, after a few months, they would finally become disgusted with me and throw me out of their homes. I used and lost many good friends that way.

I was eventually convinced to return for another psychiatric hospitalization, on this occasion, to a unit with open bathroom doors so I could be observed at all times. Again, seemingly highly motivated, I used on the unit, in spite of my best intentions, and was caught smuggling in more drugs. Embarrassed by the humiliating strip-search and discovery, I left the unit but somehow managed to stay clean outside, through sheer determination and supportive friends, long enough to land a job at a plasma center.

I didn't last long. In the process of setting up the clinic, I ordered Talwin for the "crash cart" and managed to rapidly deplete the supply single-handedly. I was paid a visit by the corporate medical director who had become suspicious of my overqualification combined with my overuse of the restroom. He was not impressed.

I returned to living off friends. Borrowing cars and sleeping on sofas, I had become a derelict. For anyone else I suppose this would represent a bottom and then the only path would be up. Unfortunately, I still had the wherewithal to continue obtaining drugs. I still had a medical license and good credit. Friendly pharmacists would fill my orders for "office use." Failing that, I would write prescriptions for mythical patients and pick them up myself, frequently paying with credit cards.

Driven by a primal instinct for survival, if nothing else, I managed to get clean again, long enough to gather myself up and get a new job, a car and a place of my own. I started working in a large clinic in an impoverished area of town and started a new career in family practice. A week or so after starting there, I returned to the use of drugs but somehow managed to appear normal enough to escape suspicion. Because of my shortcomings, I attempted to overcompensate by being the friendliest, wisest, most competent, well-read, and compassionate physician at the clinic. I did well, in spite of the drugs, and eventually was asked to head the peer review committee. How ironic! Reviewing the quality of my colleagues' practice when I was the most despicable of the lot.

My awareness vacillated between full-blown denial and, in occasional moments of clarity, a startling realization that I had deteriorated to the lowest level of human existence. I felt like a slug, a tapeworm, a repulsive parasite of the meanest order. I could not look at myself in a mirror or honestly contemplate the disgusting condition in which I had found myself.

Abandonment of Hope

The delusion that I was functioning well was exploded by a singular occurrence. I developed an allergy to Talwin. At first, rather insidiously, the drug that appeared to be my sustenance turned on me. Swelling and bruises gave way to frank ulcerations. Assuming an allergy, I tried antihistamines to no avail. Out of desperation, I tried Decadron, a potent form of cortisone, which seemed to do the trick. A temporary solution to a temporary (I thought) problem, as I planned to stop for good "tomorrow." But tomorrow never seemed to come, and I continued my insane behavior for five more years. I subsequently suffered the consequences of chronic cortisone use as well.

Given time, the Decadron lost its effect and the skin ulceration continued. Certainly one of the most insane acts is to repeatedly do something and expect different results. Each time I injected, I hoped and prayed that "this time it will be different," or I justified it with "this is the last time." But nothing changed, the results were always the same, and it never appeared to be the last time.

My condition got progressively worse: I was succumbing to the effects of the cortisone, with physical as well as psychological deterioration, and my arms and legs were covered with draining sores. As my mental processes deteriorated, I quit my job and tried to heal myself while holding up alone in my apartment. I felt too embarrassed at what I had done to myself to seek professional help. Besides, it had not seemed to work in the past. Withdrawing to my cave to lick my wounds, I decided to start taking antidepressants, since I felt more hopeless and lost than ever. They only succeeded in making me more toxic and delirious, and in that state I made a decision to end it all.

I carefully planned my demise, made sure everyone thought I was out of town, tidied up a few loose ends, and took five times the lethal dose of chloral hydrate (a sleeping pill), washing it down with red creme soda, and calmly went to bed. It was gloriously peaceful.

God, however, apparently had other plans for me. Jeannie, my fiancee, thirty miles away, had a sudden premonition that something was wrong. Without a car, she convinced a neighbor to drive her through a blinding rainstorm in the middle of the night to my place and roust the manager out of his bed to open my apartment. Paramedics rushed me to a local hospital, where I spent the next four days in a coma. (I remain in awe at the peculiar psychic connection that resulted in my rescue that night.)

After I came to, I was transferred out of the ICU to a private room. After settling in, I called a local outside pharmacy for some

Talwin to be delivered to my hospital room. It seemed like a good idea at the time; however, my treating physician did not agree, and instead of a "care package" arriving, several men in white coats came in and strapped me to a gurney for a short trip to a nearby, locked psychiatric unit and thirty more days of institutionalization.

My physical wounds healed; and, somewhat emotionally restored, I was sent home to Jeannie's on more antidepressants. It took several months to bounce back this time, and I felt that I was done with my addiction. I could not imagine myself ever using drugs again and running the risk of returning to the insanity, humiliation and degradation from whence I had come.

I began working as a physician for a religious organization. It seemed the perfect solution: an impossibly bad person like me surrounded by wonderful, charismatic, religious people could not possibly get into trouble. The proper environment was the solution. But it didn't work for long; all the collective spirituality of these fine people could not protect me from myself, seemingly bent on self-destruction. The juggernaut of my addiction hurtled me to the brink of oblivion. The curious coincidence of my being rescued by my fiancee with the breath of life still in me seemed for naught, a cruel jest of fate. (I later learned that "coincidence" is defined as God working anonymously.)

I managed to "control" my use for a while and went back to work at the clinic. Things eventually got worse, as would be expected. I finally left and after failing again at home, entered a health farm in Hawaii. By this time, still on cortisone, I was quite swollen and edematous. With a steady diet of rabbit food and bird seed, and regular jogging, I lost some of the weight and felt physically stronger (in spite of a few clandestine trips to McDonald's and the local pharmacy for occasional Talwin).

Refreshed and rejuvenated, I returned to San Diego and entered into a group practice with four other doctors. Things appeared to be going better and for the first time in seven years, I was confining my use to one day out of the week, convincing myself that I was in control. With things looking up, I married Jeannie, assuming that the added responsibilities of marriage and family would keep me on the straight and narrow. For her part, Jeannie began perceiving me in relative terms, and indeed I appeared to be doing better.

Eventually, I reverted to my old habits of continually using throughout the day, and my practice began to falter. My partners, one by one, began to drop out of the practice or move out of town and my patient load dwindled. Could it be that my falling asleep while taking histories or frequently excusing myself for an unusually lengthy visit to the restroom aroused suspicion? In the meantime, I was physically deteriorating. I had a large ulceration on my left arm, which became infected with subsequent erosion and loss of tendons and bone. The necrotic lesion was noticeably malodorous, and I feared everyone knew what was happening. I feared the worst.

Recovery Begins

Fortunately, the "worst" did occur. I was paid a visit by a Drug Enforcement Administration (DEA) investigator who was concerned about the amount of Talwin I was ordering "for office use." It seems that in the course of auditing one of the *seven* pharmacies that was supplying me, they noticed an inordinate amount signed out to my office. The agent was kind enough to not make any accusations but instead gave me a phone number in Sacramento of the Physicians' Diversion Program. As he left, he stated he would be back to follow up on how I was doing.

Trembling, with visions of losing everything and being sodomized in prison dancing in my head, I made the call which subsequently saved my life.

Unknown to me at the time, the California state licensing board had made a significant change in policy to establish the Diversion Program. Formerly, punitive action was taken with loss of license and criminal charges, as appropriate. They now had decided that it was more cost-effective to attempt to salvage physicians by treating chemical dependency problems rather than shooting their wounded, as had been the case. This novel approach had just been placed into action in 1980, the year in which they had intervened with me.

When I met with the Diversion Evaluation Committee, they "suggested" I shut down my practice and enter a chemical dependency program at Sharp-Cabrillo Hospital in San Diego. I had no options left at this point but to follow directions.

At this juncture, I began experiencing the process of surrender. I had no will left to fight as I had been doing over the previous ten years. I feared this was the end—I was going out with a whimper. I had so wanted to conquer my addiction on my own but had been unable to do so. I felt totally defeated and demoralized when I entered that hospital.

Through the fog of despair, a few rays of hope broke. For the first time in all my treatment experiences, I was treated by doctors who themselves had had problems with addiction. I had formerly been taught that I was using drugs to self-medicate an underlying psychiatric condition. On this occasion, however, I was told I had used drugs because I was a drug addict—a rather novel concept. All the emphasis over the past years had been placed on treating my neuroses while overlooking my primary disease: addiction.

A good deal of the initial treatment was aimed at physical problems. On admission, as a result of five years of taking Decadron, I was edematous and obese, weighing 207 pounds and unable to wear my usual shoes or clothing. I also had a large open wound on my left forearm with exposed, infected bone. The first ten days of my treatment involved detoxification from the narcotics, local wound treatment, and biopsy of the bone, which appeared cancerous on the x-rays. After I was pronounced reasonably medically stable, I was thrown into rehabilitation treatment with a motley variety of folks with whom I felt I had little in common. Initially, I felt out of place—somehow different from these people who I recognized as alcoholics and addicts. I did not fit the stereotype and felt I had little to gain from the treatment experience. The educational material was of interest and fine for "those" people, but I could not see how it all applied to me. With time, the fog began to lift, and some of it began to make sense to me.

My first hurdle was the overwhelming sense of shame and guilt at what I had done and the depths to which I had sunk. Two little phrases that I learned there aided in my deliverance from the bondage of guilt: "He retaineth not His anger forever, because He delighteth in mercy," and "God has absolutely no attitude of condemnation toward man." Armed with these, I could now set about learning to forgive myself and later seeking the forgiveness of those who I had harmed. I learned that I had a disease, primary and hereditary; my addiction was not a case of moral turpitude from which I could have extricated myself with a little willpower and a good pull on the bootstraps. I was taught that I was not responsible for my disease, but that I was responsible for my recovery. Thus, much of the emphasis in treatment was not on the problem, but rather on the solution. I was told to stop asking "Why?" and begin instead to seek the answers to the question "How?"

I found the group therapy to be very much different than what I had been used to in psychiatric facilities. We avoided intellectual discussions and focused strictly on feelings. I had been anaesthetized for so long, I did not have a clue as to what I was feeling at any given time. Much of my treatment revolved around learning to identify basic feelings with which I had lost touch long ago.

During my first outside excursion, two weeks after arriving, my eyes were treated to a feast of a hillside covered with golden poppies. It was as if I had been seeing in black and white and my world had suddenly changed to Technicolor. Subtle changes in my perceptions and emotions, although seemingly minor, became events of great rejoicing. Little by little, some degree of hope was invading my spirit.

I made friends in treatment with others who came from varied backgrounds and belief systems. The common bond of our disease brought us, out of desperation, as close as the passengers on a sinking ship. This degree of desperation and loneliness are only known to the dying. Initially we need someone with whom to share our pain and fear; they later become the partners in our joy. It became clear to me that I could not recover alone because my disease thrives on solitude.

While in the hospital we were bussed out to local meetings of Alcoholics Anonymous and Narcotics Anonymous. My experience with the former was one of distant affection, initially feeling that it was wonderful for "those" alcoholics. I looked forward to my first N.A. meeting, but it was less rewarding than I had expected. All I seemed to notice in the meeting, as I self-righteously gazed about, were those who had Mohawk haircuts, wore leather and chains, or looked as though they had been sleeping under bridges for the better part of their lives. Fortunately, I was forced to attend meetings every night and slowly began to put away my prejudices and listen. I began hearing my own story and related to the feelings. Here, after all, was a group of people, on the outside, that could do what I had never been able to do—stay clean. And, I later realized, I probably didn't look too good to them at that point either. Yet some were kind enough to hug me in spite of my despicable appearance.

Going Home

The day came when I was to go home. I faced discharge with some degree of trepidation since I felt safe in a supportive environment. It had been recommended that I go to a treatment center in Georgia, specializing in physicians, for extended residential treatment, but financial distress precluded that and I had to go out and face the world which I had left. It had not changed; my only hope was that I had.

It had also been suggested that I take a brief hiatus from the practice of medicine and instead direct all my energies at developing and maintaining my recovery. The hospital stay was only a beginning and, as I was told, the real recovery is "out there." I had been introduced to the local recovering community while in treatment, and upon leaving the hospital became actively involved with others who had tread this path before me. I found there were scores of people similar to me in their plight and eager to help me along the path of recovery.

I perceive recovery as a journey, much like Bunyan's Pilgrim experienced; the path is full of snares and potholes arising out of my own fears, prejudices, and insecurities. I, too, feared the lions on the road to Mount Zion, and my faith tested the mettle of their chains. This journey, however, has no completion, unless it is in the final repose; it is continuous, the road ever changing. And, like the Pilgrim's, those "steps may be tread with sorrow or with delight." The choice is mine.

I found that my recovering friends were a major asset in my own early recovery. They represented a vast storehouse of experience and knowledge from which I could freely benefit. At first, there were relatively few of us involved in the local fellowship of recovering drug addicts, but, with time, we grew. Initially our goal was to provide a meeting each night for support of those, like myself, who were seeking recovery from drug addiction. But somehow it all snowballed over the course of six years and became larger than we could have foreseen. At this time, there are over one hundred thirty groups meeting weekly in San Diego County. Expansion has occurred on the international level as well, and now drug addicts in forty countries around the world have the opportunity to recover with the same program. A startling accomplishment for a few drug addicts—former ne'er-do-wells—armed with no creed or dogma other than the common belief that recovery should be available to anyone seeking relief from the horrors of addiction.

I owe much of what I have today to those fine people who selflessly gave their experience, strength and hope to me in my early recovery. They only asked that I, in turn, pass it on to others, giving freely of that which was freely given to me.

In my first six months of recovery, I was honored to be a contributor to a textbook on recovery, written "by committee," that has so far sold half a million copies. Initially, I felt inadequate and ill-prepared, but with the encouragement of friends, I realized that I had something to share in my overcoming my feelings of uniqueness. It made me feel as if I had played a small role in thousands of others' recoveries and gave me some feeling of worth and pride in my own.

Challenges and unforeseen rewards have become the rule for me. I had fears that life without drugs would be dull and boring, but instead have found the opposite to be the case. This has been the most exciting and challenging portion of my life. I have found the wonders of the universe laid at my feet, and, like Newton, "the vast ocean of truth lying undiscovered before me."

As long as my primary focus is on my spiritual growth, all other aspects of my life seem to fall in order. Material and financial matters have fallen into place to the exact extent that they continue to remain secondary priorities. I have been freed from the fears that once controlled my motivation and actions. I have become comfortable with who and what I am. I no longer regret the past or live in fear of what the future may hold for me. I have found how my experiences, no matter how degrading, can benefit others. I have found my place in the universe and my life has become simplified with precise boundaries when I have relinquished my position of (seeming) control over other people and things. The solutions to seemingly impossible problems always come. My life has taken on new meaning and new direction and I feel that if I were to die today, I would have died a success knowing that I have accomplished something positive in this short lifetime.

My family life has likewise improved; in part due to abstinence alone, but much repair work had to be done to my relationship with Jeannie. It was surprising that we had weathered the storm together but the real challenge was in the rebuilding.

Early in our relationship, I don't believe Jeannie was aware of the extent of my disease. Even if she occasionally was wont to catch glimpses of its horrors, it may have been easier to deny the obvious and believe something else to be the case. She apparently saw something positive in me, through the haze of my addiction, because she believed in me and had faith that there was a solution to this nightmare, which at times must have appeared overwhelming. I had made many heroic attempts at stopping on my own and she believed in my sincerity and had faith that God would bring about an ultimate victory for us. Many times, I must have shattered those beliefs with relapses, but she still held out for a solution in spite of the seeming setbacks. Supporting me through those bleak times with only love and a little faith separating us from the brink of the abyss was the challenge of her life.

I would not have blamed her if she had made her exit during one of those seemingly hopeless times, but she stubbornly held on with superhuman strength, which constantly reinforced my courage. I believe wives should receive medals for their ability to tenaciously hold on through the worst of crises when surely most of us men would have left long before.

While I was in the hospital, Jeannie attended all the treatment activities and gained some significant degree of hope long before I could see any chance for my own recovery. Her constant encouragement was my only source of strength early on and I cannot thank her enough for that. We were both told that couples rarely made it through these crises intact, and I suppose that served to encourage us to try all the harder.

Jeannie made coffee and acted as hostess for our innumerable gatherings of recovering people. She made wall decorations and floral arrangements for tables at dances and other social activities we hosted to provide a drug-free social life for ourselves and others trying to recover. She was supportive without being overbearing or watchful. The realization that I could return to active addiction at any time was there, but she had let go and allowed me the freedom I needed at that time.

About a year into my recovery, we received word that the stork was planning a visit in the near future—a welcome gift for those of us returning to the realm of the living. I was beside myself, strutting about like a peacock with the relief that my virility had been restored (so much so that it had overcome the modern scientific methods of birth control).

There was, of course, some fear surrounding this blessed event. We did not feel financially stable enough at the time and I had some misgivings about my own abilities to be an effective parent. My two stepchildren, Andy and Trayce, grew up in the shadow of my active addiction and I felt I had failed them. I had succeeded only in distancing myself from them and creating barriers between us. Without actively abusing them, I was guilty of emotional neglect. Fearing I had nothing to offer them in the way of a positive role model, I withdrew into my cocoon of self-loathing.

If we had had our way, we may have waited for "better times," but God had a different plan and His timing proved to be better. The arrival of Katie-Beth gave me an opportunity to take on a new role in life and learn new tasks. The experience of her birth was a startling affirmation of the wonders of God's universe. I felt much like a small child mesmerized by the heavens on a starlit night. It all seemed so vast and wonderful, beyond my ken. I had delivered many children myself, but the arrival of this special gift was particularly miraculous to me as I examined her thoroughly in the delivery room and basked in the glory of her perfection. She was intact and bore none of the stigmata of my former life. She was an affirmation of recovery.

As I am still a child in my own recovery, I only have two years on my daughter Katie-Beth. The beauty of it is that she never knew her father as a drug addict. She has grown up in a stable environment, now for four years, and has never had to experience the confusion of an unpredictable, usually absent father. She represents a very special divine gift to me, and is, and will continue to be, spoiled rotten.

Knowing what I do about the genetic nature of my disease, people ask me if I fear that Katie-Beth will follow in my footsteps. She may indeed be prone to addiction, but I know that the disease is in fact immensely treatable and maybe even preventable given the proper education. She will have a chance to learn at a young age, that which I could only learn after experiencing years of hopelessness and despair.

Another Test

During my first year of recovery, much effort was made toward restoring my physical health. After detoxification from the narcotics, I was slowly weaned off the Decadron and subsequently lost thirty pounds of weight. During that period, I had a flair-up of psoriasis necessitating more aggressive treatment of that as well. The fear of cancer of the bone was dispelled by a biopsy that revealed osteomyelitis, an infection in the bone and surrounding tissue. I underwent vigorous antibiotic therapy and subsequently several reconstructive surgical procedures, and I now have relatively good function of my left arm. (At one point a recommendation had been made for amputation.) I was very grateful to be as physically restored as I was, but the greater miracle was that I never had to take any narcotics during that period (or since).

The disease of addiction is never cured. It can be arrested but lays dormant until retriggered by exposure to drugs. By this time, I had learned to cherish the little bit of recovery I had, and consequently looked upon surgery and possible exposure to narcotics with some degree of trepidation. I knew one of my greatest faults lay in the belief system of "justified" use of narcotics. When I needed surgery, I could not have asked for a more justifiable reason for the use of narcotics; I knew I should not be a foolish martyr just for the sake of abstinence. On the other hand, I knew also that my brain could not distinguish the effect of the drug regardless of the source or indication. Once a narcotic was in my system, that horrible monster lying dormant in my brain would be loosed and I could not guarantee my actions.

I discussed my concerns with the professionals involved in my case as well as members of my support group. Because of the extent of the surgery, my surgeon felt compelled to write a post-op order for Demerol and I was encouraged to take it as needed. Members of my support group helped me prepare myself emotionally and spiritually, dealing with fear and self-pity, the two components of pain that can exaggerate its experience and convert physiological pain into suffering. Having prepared myself, I felt at peace prior to surgery and the subsequent events proved to be tolerable.

On awakening from the anaesthetic, I instinctively reached for the nurses' call button and awaited the inevitable pain. The effect of the anaesthetic alone had altered my thinking. I became obsessed with drugs again. Deliriously, the wheels of the more primitive portions of my mind began turning again and I began making plans for the Demerol. I had an intravenous line in my neck, and began wondering how long it would take to reach my brain if I could convince the nurse to administer it via that route. I seemed to have no control over the obsessive thoughts, and experienced the return of that incredible compulsion to use drugs in spite of the consequences.

The miracle, though, was more powerful though than my craving. I laid for some time waiting for the inevitable pain so I could justify asking for the Demerol, but for some reason it never came. I laid there in the hospital for three days, secretly hoping for a twinge of pain, but was denied and consequently spared the horror of the return of my addiction.

I can only believe it was divine intervention because I have never been very stoic or capable of handling pain. In this case I didn't have to try and grit my teeth and bear it; there just wasn't any pain. I know if I had had the slightest provocation, I would have rewarded myself with chemical surcease without hesitation. My only explanation is that God was more aware of my disease at that point than I could have been, and was aware that even a small amount of "justified" narcotic would have been disastrous.

A Career Reborn

The Diversion Committee, besides their involvement initially, fairly insisted that I not return to medical practice in early abstinence, but use that time to further my own personal recovery in addition to pursuing the ongoing medical treatment I required. Initial fears that my career was doomed evaporated with time. Things couldn't have worked out better, but lacking the patience and faith that come with recovery, the early months were filled with insecurities. With extra time on my hands, I began volunteering at the hospital where I had gone through treatment. Initially helping out where I could, I later began running study groups and facilitating aftercare workshops. After a year, I was asked to join the staff as a half-time physician. I must admit I was elated to have been asked to work with physicians who I held in high esteem and in a field which fascinated me. However, I faced my new appointment with some degree of dread.

It had been one and a half years since I had practiced medicine, and then only loaded. What if I had forgotten everything or could I even practice medicine without drugs in my system? Again, my fears were for naught. The art of medicine, like riding a bicycle, returned to me and indeed proved to be very different in that it was a vast improvement over my previous practice. I could now empathize with all my patients and my experience became a common ground on which my patients and I could bond.

I found that I had much to learn. Although I had spent some years practicing my own addiction, it was a far different thing to know how to treat it. I became obsessed with learning everything there was to know about the field. There were no standard textbooks or training courses, so I found and read everything else I could get my hands on, from esoteric scientific journals to self-help group pamphlets. I picked other people's brains shamelessly and joined professional societies of those in the field. After several years of further education (primarily self-taught) I had an opportunity to sit for a certification exam and become duly certified as an "addictionologist." I have since become involved with the certification committee and help make up exam questions for other physicians seeking certification in the field.

My career has continued to flourish. Seemingly born out of the ashes of my previous professional life, I have had opportunities continuously arise to expand my work. Although primarily involved with the medical treatment of the chemically dependent, I have become a consultant to a variety of educational, treatment, and law enforcement groups, including the DEA, the agency that initially investigated my (self-)prescribing practices.

After completing over three years of monitoring by the Physicians' Diversion Program, I became a graduate consultant to that body. I have had a variety of opportunities to work with other physicians who have been caught up in the same whirlpool as I. We are a particularly difficult group, on the whole, with which to deal, but the satisfaction of seeing even one physician return to active practice and healthily recovering is without parallel.

Gaining some degree of notoriety in the field of chemical dependency, I have found myself in a unique position to serve that very large population of people who are suffering from this disease. My primary focus has been in the clinical practice of medicine, but I find myself more and more involved in educating the public. I seem to get more requests than I can honor to speak to various civic and educational groups. I lecture at several of the local colleges and universities which are now beginning to offer curricula in the field. I have been asked to visit several foreign countries to help set up treatment centers and have even become embroiled in some of their local politics. Not perceiving myself as a political activist, I felt uncomfortable in that role, but I cannot doubt the need for someone to act as an advocate for those afflicted with the disease of addiction.

I have met here with visiting foreign dignitaries who are seeking solutions for their local problems and have become very excited about the prospects of introducing modern therapeutics to other, less fortunate areas of the globe that are likewise plagued with chemical dependency issues and currently foundering in the quagmire of ignorance and intolerance.

It seems at times that I have taken on more than I can possibly handle. More needs arise that are not being met and I have a difficult time turning my back on them. It seems I have become as obsessed with the treatment of addiction as I was with drugs not so long ago. Life would be simpler if I limited my work, but when I appreciate the gratitude I have for my own personal recovery, then I realize I owe a large debt to society as a whole and especially those who are touched by this disease. I now know why I spent so many years in unspeakable torment while actively dependent on narcotics. It qualified me for that noble calling which I sought when I went to medical school. I had to pay my dues before I could be of service to others who are still suffering.

I have received so much in my recovery and now realize that everything I have is through grace (i.e., an unearned gift). Since it has all been so freely given to me, it is incumbent upon me to freely give to those, less fortunate than I, who are seeking a way out of the maelstrom of addiction. I have followed a rather circuitous route, but have gained that noble purpose and those noble virtues to which I had aspired years ago.

The more I have grown in my own recovery, the more grateful I have become for being born with this disease of drug addiction. When looking at the horrors and utter despair of my former life, one would be hard pressed to comprehend a feeling of gratitude, yet I know I would have never experienced the joys of recovery or have had the opportunity to serve others as I do today without first having walked that tortuous and rocky road of living death.

Not long ago I observed a sign in a church youth hall stating: "What you are is God's gift to you—what you make of yourself is your gift to God." I thought how true that was of me, for God's gift was my addiction, and my recovery is my gift to Him and my fellow man. Through my addiction and my subsequent recovery, I have found a new direction and a new purpose for my life. I have the opportunity to practice the noblest of professions: that of service to my afflicted fellow man. There is no higher calling.

SUICIDE

About the Author

In her late teens and twenties, Janet Jacobsen obsessed about death in the same way that her peers may have about dating or appearance. She dreamed of elaborate ways of killing herself, idolized people who had died, and could think of no reason for living. She became addicted to having suicidal thoughts, which gave her a kind of "high" and an escape from daily pressures.

She attempted suicide numerous times, once resulting in a coma, followed by involuntary confinement in a mental institution. Although she tried various types of therapy, she continued to find refuge in the knowledge that she could take her own life.

Janet Jacobsen stopped pursuing suicide more than ten years ago. She has a firm commitment to self-awareness and maintaining a positive attitutde in all phases of her life. She supports herself as a successful artist and craftsperson, and helps others through peer counseling and the practice of Intuitive Massage.

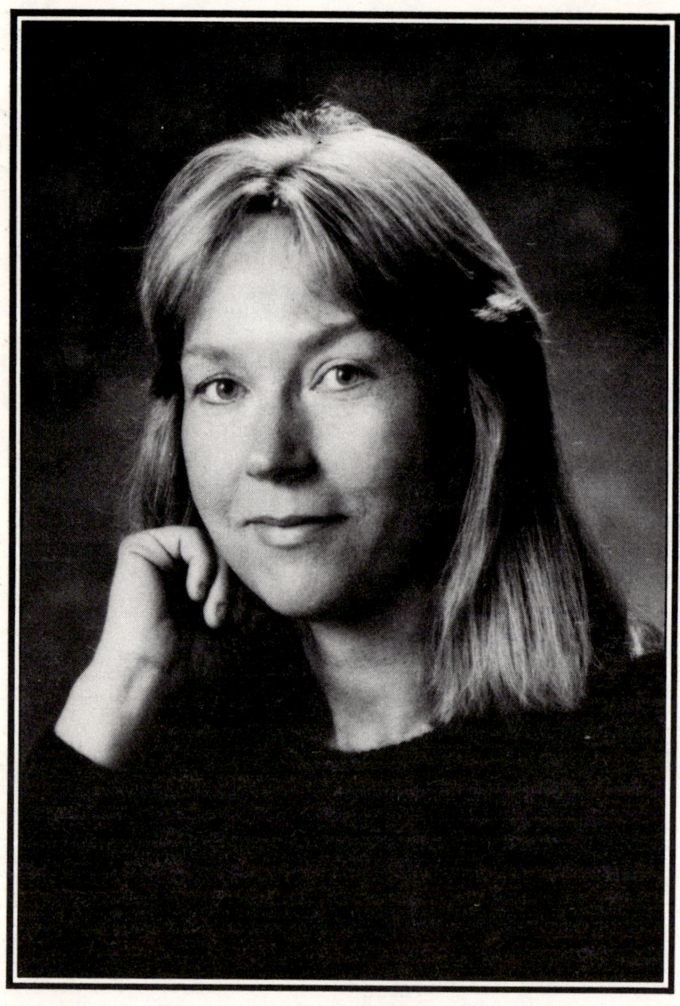

Janet Jacobsen

Killing the Pain

by
Janet Jacobsen

****

My Niece, Myself

I've been thinking about suicide a lot lately. Not because I want to kill myself, although for ten years of my life I was obsessed with an urge to die that resulted in numerous suicide attempts and finally a coma and commitment to a mental hospital. I've been free of suicidal thoughts for over ten years now. Recently, however, I got a long distance phone call from my sixteen-year-old niece. She was drilling me with questions about the times I had overdosed on pills: What kind did I take? How many had I taken? How many would kill? How long did it take for them to take effect?

I became alarmed and asked her, "Why are you asking me this? Are you thinking about killing yourself?" There was a silence. Finally she said, "I'm taking pills right now. I've just taken 40 Tylenol."

"Why? What's wrong? Why are you doing this?"

She just said, "Now I'm up to 45."

I was frightened. She was thousands of miles away and I couldn't get to her. I had to reach her with words. I wanted to say to her what I would have wanted said to me. What would have stopped me? Instead I heard myself saying ineffectual things like, "You have so much going for you," and "There's so much to live for." But I remembered that in her state of mind there was no hope. The future could only be seen from the hopeless vantage point of the present.

I asked her, "What are you feeling right now?"

"Nothing," she replied. She sounded stoical and resolved. "Now I'm up to 50."

I thought back to one of the times she was asking me about, 16 years ago when I was 21. I had 600 aspirin in front of me and intended to take them all. What was I feeling? What was I thinking? I remember that I didn't want to chicken out, as I'd done in the past. I was afraid of going only halfway and surviving, but being brain-damaged. I also worried about the possibility of reincarnation. What if there really was such a thing and I came back even worse off?

I wanted to convince myself, to push myself through it by thinking, "I just don't fit in. I never have. I never will. I don't know what's wrong with me. I'm different from everyone. I'm too sensitive, too emotional. It hurts all the time." Aspirin was for killing pain and that's what I wanted to do, permanently.

I thought about my mother asleep in her room. She would be shocked because she knew nothing about how I was feeling right now. She had always wanted me to be happy, and if I wasn't, she didn't want to know about it. Feelings were never discussed, as if they were some dreaded disease which maybe would just go away.

I felt so alone, like I was the only one who had such dark, deep feelings inside. I knew no one could ever love me. I began to put the pills in my mouth three at a time and washed them down with a sweet, cheap wine that burned my throat. I had read that combining pills with alcohol increased the chances of fatality. I took three more pills and another swig of wine, swallowing quickly so that the aspirin wouldn't dissolve in my mouth. Three more pills, and three more. I went on and on mechanically, telling myself, "Don't think. Don't feel." It was like a dream: I wasn't fully present, I was just a body swallowing pills.

After I'd taken about 80 aspirin there was a ringing in my head that was getting louder and louder, alarming me to the reality of what I was doing. I could feel the effect on my body and I began to panic. Even though my heart was crying, "Don't stop now! Keep going! Keep going," all I could think about was maybe I would live and be brain-damaged. This thought terrified me so much that at two in the morning, I stumbled my way into my mother's room and told her what I'd done. She rushed me to the hospital and we drove in silence. I could see her anguish and she could see mine, but we didn't talk about it; we didn't know how.

At the hospital emergency room I was given a bitter liquid that made me throw up until all that came up was green bile. I was placed in intensive care and was watched carefully by the nurses in the adjoining room. I heard them talking about me, saying I had "everything to live for," and I thought they sounded disgusted that I would do such a thing. They didn't know how much I hurt, a hurt that just wouldn't go away.

I have heard many people say that they can't understand such a drastic act as suicide. But at the time it seemed to be the only thing that made sense. I had an unrelenting ache, like cancer, that was excruciatingly painful. As I think back on it I'm amazed that I could have lived that way for so long, in a constant state of physical contraction, like a vice, choking off my life's energy: breathing shallowly, holding myself in, living in the constant fear of being myself. Self-hate ate away at me like acid, until the only solution to end the suffering was death. How did it ever get so bad?

Early Childhood

I believe that from the very beginning, since infancy, I was extremely sensitive and easily hurt. My natural expressions of hurt and anger were strictly discouraged by my mother, who was frightened of strong emotions. To her, feelings meant pain, and she thought that if she could make the feelings stop, then the pain would stop. But, of course, it didn't; it just festered like an unattended, infected wound. My attempts to assert my aliveness also angered my older brother, who resented me for replacing him as baby of the family. He would exert his power over me by continually taking my bottle away and even, when I was nine months old, pushing me down a flight of stairs that I had just painstakingly crawled up to be with him.

I spent my first birthday in the hospital with pneumonia, where I was left to scream through the night every night for two weeks. My congested lungs obstructed my breathing, and I felt terrified and abandoned. I can imagine my baby self observing, "It's not safe to feel or to express. I get rejected, hurt, and sent away." I believe I decided right then to be really quiet, make myself small and take up as little space as possible. The fear of being myself was equalled by the anger that I wasn't allowed to be myself. The anger wanted to scream, "I'm here!" But the fear demanded, "Be quiet!" This hardened into a shell of deadness that protected me from feeling the deep pain of my unfulfilled longing to be held and loved for my whole real self. If I couldn't be held with love and acceptance, then I didn't want to be held at all.

I became a painfully shy child and would hide behind my mother's skirt, afraid to utter a word, make a mistake, or offend someone. I could be nothing less than perfect, and, that being impossible, I kept quiet and appeared to be sweet and unassuming. But stuffed feelings were continually threatening to pop out like angry Jack-in-the-boxes until finally the pressure was so great that feelings seeped out in a scowling moodiness and I was proclaimed "ugly" and "bad" by a mother who preferred that there be only pleasantness at all costs. "What's wrong with you?" she would ask. I was caught on this pendulum for years, swinging between fear and anger, being a good girl and a bad girl, a wimp and a witch, until eventually, years later, this escalated to the extremes of a zombie-like deadness which could only be relieved by adrenalized acts of self-destruction.

My dad and I had similar temperaments and I adored him. He was artistic and so was I, and he praised me for my art work. But when I was seven, my sister was born, and he shifted his attention from me to her. I felt like I'd been abandoned again. I felt hurt and angry and unimportant. Losing the attention of my father caused a pain so deep that I started overeating to numb it. I came to the conclusion that I couldn't win, I wasn't good enough, and I always lost what I cared about, so I decided that I wouldn't let myself care. I remember one day, when I was eight, I saw my father fall down a flight of stairs and hurt his back. A little neighbor boy ran to him full of concern, but I just stood there watching and wondering why I didn't feel anything.

One time, years later, on Father's Day, when he was presented with a cake and some gifts, he broke down crying, saying, "Nobody cares about me, nobody loves me." I had never seen him cry before and didn't know he had the same pain I had. I spontaneously put my arms around him. Crying I said, "I love you, Daddy." I hadn't hugged him since I was a little girl. But he was uncomfortable and brusquely pushed me away. I was deeply hurt and strongly resolved to never let myself be vulnerable like that again.

As the years passed, I developed a philosophy that said, "Think negatively, then if you don't get what you want you won't be disappointed, and if you do, you'll be happily surprised." There were very few happy surprises. One day at school, when I was 14, we combined the male and female gym classes to learn square dancing. The boys were instructed to come over to the girls' side and pick a partner. Being shy and pudgy and virtually invisible, I was terrified that no one would ask me to dance. One by one I saw the other girls being asked, until I began to realize that I was going to be left alone without a partner. I panicked and bolted out of there and hid in the locker room, ashamed. Nobody wanted me. I couldn't bear the humiliation. I was afraid that probably no one would ever want me.

Changing Self Images

I felt I had to do something and became intent upon making myself noticeable and desirable. I spent all my time fantasizing, imagining myself as slim and pretty, seeing boys wanting me. As these fantasies occupied my nights, my days were spent losing weight, letting my blonde hair grow long and straight, learning how to apply makeup, and buying clothes that were tight-fitting and sexy. Marilyn Monroe was my idol and I wanted to be like her. The whole effect pleaded, "Look at me! Notice me!" It worked. I was no longer invisible. I had created a new identity.

I was thrilled with the attention I was getting. One girl told me, "Last year no one knew who you were. This year the whole school knows." I had gone from nonentity to notorious. I now smoked cigarettes and drank alcohol, which made me feel less inhibited. I even shoplifted a few times. Once, I was caught and arrested, while just the week before I had written and delivered a sermon in front of my church congregation, representing my Bible class. I felt like a "bad girl," but it was a lot better than being a "quiet girl," It was more fun. I felt alive.

An older boy of 18 started to take an interest in me. He was handsome and cool and he wanted me. We began seeing each other and in the few weeks that we dated I became infatuated with him. I was hungry for the attention he gave me and I felt an excitement that I had never felt before. Then, suddenly, he stopped calling and I found out that he'd gone back to his old girlfriend. He didn't want me. I was alone again. I had let myself care, and now I was devastated. "I lose whatever I care about." It hurt so much that for the first time I began to wish I were dead. I became obsessed with the thought of walking out in front of a car. I sat in my room imagining the scene, seeing how in one crushing blow it would all be over. This was the only way I could think of to make the pain go away.

I tried to forget him by going to dances. At one of these I was asked to slow dance by a nice-looking boy. He held me close and I felt desirable again. Then another boy cut in on him, and then another boy. It was quite a change from the 14-year-old me who was unnoticed. As more and more boys cut in, I could see them clustered together on the side of the dance floor, laughing and pointing at me. They were just using me—it was a game to them. This was as humiliating as being invisible. Either way I felt worthless.

Even though I had the appearance of being sexy and loose, a strict sense of morality had never let me go beyond kissing. Yet, I began to hear rumors about me. I'd walk down the hall at school and boys would whistle and make lewd comments. My reputation as a "bad girl" was snowballing and boys I had never even talked to were saying that they'd slept with me. I thought of Marilyn Monroe, who had recently committed suicide, and I understood how she must have felt. It hurt to be seen only as an object to ridicule and joke about, just as much as it had hurt to not be seen at all. I wondered why I couldn't just be appreciated as a person?

At 17, I desperately tried to undo my bad reputation and erase my sexy image. I began to wear conservative clothes and walk in a straightforward way. I became an "A" student, had my writings published in the school literary magazine and won awards for my high grades. I was a good girl again. When I was a "good girl" I felt quiet, dulled, and invisible. When I was a "bad girl" I felt expressive, but judged and ridiculed. I didn't know any in-between way of being, and I hated both these selves. In the tunnel vision of this negative mind-set, I could only see what was bad about my life, until all I could think of was how much I wanted it to be over.

A biology teacher at school had told us that if we didn't urinate for 18 hours, it would secrete back into the bloodstream and we would die. I played with that idea for awhile. What would it be like if I were dead? I imagined people being sorry that they hadn't been nicer to me, and I visualized them weeping at my funeral. I couldn't ask for their concern in life; I could only imagine it in death.

One night I went to bed with that plan in mind. I hadn't gone to the bathroom since five o'clock that night and I figured that by eleven o'clock the next morning (if I didn't wet the bed), I would be dead. The means were uncertain, but the intention was clear.

At one in the morning, I was awakened by my mother screaming my name over and over. I thought something terrible must have happened. It had. I went fearfully into her bedroom and saw my father lying on the floor, dead. He had suffered a fatal heart attack. The night I had intended to die, he had died instead. I was shocked. I didn't believe it was a coincidence. Did he go instead of me? Did he die so I could live?

I had loved him so dearly as a little girl but had not been close to him since my sister had been born. My hurt had hardened around me into a protective wall of resentment towards him and I barely spoke to him.

He'd been an excitable man, often exploding into anger, and I'd been afraid of his volatility. He had the same intensity of emotion that I feared and judged in myself. He would often rage, "You'll be sorry when I'm dead!" Sometimes I'd wished that he were. And now he was. I was stunned out of my plan, but I didn't feel a deep sense of grief at his death. My brother had moved away a year earlier and it was peaceful now without their raging tempers constantly erupting.

On June 6, 1968, a year and a half later, Bobby Kennedy was killed. I was 19 and worked as a clerk-typist at the Navy Base near my home, and his death affected me so deeply I couldn't function at work. This seemed like a delayed, displaced reaction to my father's death, and I felt the grief that I wouldn't let myself feel then. I cried all day and finally had to leave work. I drove around aimlessly, crying and anguishing over the reasons for life and death, asking for answers from a God I wasn't sure existed. I walked into a store and there, in the middle of the aisle, was a large display for the book *A Search for the Truth* by Ruth Montgomery. I bought and read it and was profoundly affected as it opened up a whole new way of seeing life that made sense to me. She talked about how we are here on Earth to work on our soul development so that we can be one with God again, and how there is an "after life" where we go when we die, or "pass over," where we assess our progress and what we've learned from our Earth experience. These ideas were exciting to me and I was compelled to read more books on the "after life," reincarnation, and psychic development. I also began to read books about the "power of thought," and how our attitude affects our experience of reality. This made sense to me and I could see how my attitude of negativity had formed around me like a straitjacket and was controlling me. But at the same time I was unable and unwilling to be free of it. I didn't feel strong enough to fight the current that was sweeping me along. The "after life" that I read about seemed like a much better place than my Earth life and I longed to go to it.

Russian Roulette

I no longer cared much about my looks and ate lots of sweets—they numbed my anxiety. My cocoon was thickening around me. Within that cocoon the constant thought of death had become my preoccupation and my recreation. For hours at a time I painted portraits of those who had died: Marilyn Monroe, my dad, Bobby and John Kennedy. I also wrote poems that expressed my longing to be free from my body, "this prison of flesh."

I was still 19, and it was about that time that Helen, a high school friend, came to live with us for a year. She had injured herself falling down a flight of stairs, and my mother took her in as one of the family. She was subject to depression and black moods, and we brought that out in one another. In the room we shared, we talked about suicide the way other girls talked about clothes. We compared our death fantasies. She would tell me about the urge she had to drive off a cliff. My ideal death scenario was to fall asleep in the snow and drift off painlessly into a permanent sleep. She thought it would be great to do time-lapse photography of a corpse decaying and to drive a hearse.

Eventually, Helen moved away and I was alone again. I withdrew more and more into my secret, separate world. A sense of unreality began to blanket me, and I started to seriously think of ways to kill myself. Ironically, I felt the most alive when I was confronted with the impending possibility of death. Energy would surge through me at the thought. Fear. Adrenaline. Drama. It rattled the cage of my repressed feelings. The thought of suicide also became a comfort in a way: no matter how bad things got, I'd think, "I can always kill myself." Any other problem was trivialized by that thought. When faced with death, what else mattered? What could be worse? It was the panacea that soothed all my fears, anxieties, and hurts. But the obsessive thinking of death built to the point where I was compelled to take some kind of self-destructive action. I started to experiment with a series of mini-stabs at death.

One such time I lay in bed with a towel beneath my left wrist as I held a razor blade poised above a vein. The fear of pain and blood was excruciating, but so was the pain of my life. I slashed tentatively at my wrist until blood began to trickle out, at which point my fear of blood won and I stopped. Another time I swallowed 60 of my mother's thyroid pills, but nothing happened. A week later I swallowed ten Compoze (an over-the-counter tranquilizer) plus ten aspirin, downing them with alcohol, and fell asleep on my bed. When I awoke the next morning I was disappointed that I was still alive. Then I remembered I'd dreamt that I died but was sent back with the words, "You're not through yet. You have work to do."

I never considered leaving a suicide note for the same reason that I hid my diary and wrote in it in shorthand—I didn't want anyone to know how I felt; my feelings were what I thought was wrong with me. But, finally, at age 19, I was so frightened by my obsessive thoughts of suicide and how they were leading to more and more serious attempts, that I told my mother. She was shocked and concerned. Part of me wanted her to reach out and hold me, but because I hadn't been held by her since infancy, I think I would have pulled away in discomfort. I was afraid of what I wanted most. Maybe she was, too. But she reached out to me the best way she knew how, by finding a psychiatrist for me to see on a weekly basis.

I felt relieved that my suicidal thoughts were in the open and that help was on the way. I was happy that friends and family were concerned about me, and I no longer felt so isolated and alone. I was visible once again. I saw the psychiatrist weekly and during my sessions I intellectualized about why I was depressed and why I thought I should die. But I never let myself feel. Finally, after 6 months, he told me that my depression was actually inverted rage. I was amazed. I had always thought of it as being so passive. He helped me realize that suicide was really an aggressive, angry act. I'd never yelled or cried out loud. I silently held my feelings inside and, like a raging fire with nowhere to go, they burned me alive until the intensity of the pain demanded something equally intense to stop it—death, suicide.

For the first time, with my doctor's encouragement, I let myself feel how angry I was at my mother for not letting me express my feelings, for never admitting she had feelings, for her moral perfectionism that was critical of behavior that was less than perfect. My fire was now raging outwardly for everyone to see, and though I felt more alive than I had in years, I didn't like this self—this was the ugliness that I'd always feared and hidden. I wondered why everyone else seemed so cool and unemotional (especially my doctor), while I was filled with raging emotions. I still felt different and worse than other people. Sometimes I wondered if I was insane. When I confronted my mother with the reasons for my anger, she couldn't understand. She was sorry that I was suffering, but she insisted that I'd been born this way. That just reopened my "something's wrong with me" wound that I was trying to heal, and I felt all the more frustrated and angry.

It was uncomfortable living at home, feeling the way I did about my mother. Eventually I decided to take a big risk. A girl I worked with told me that she'd always been shy and unhappy and how going to Hawaii had completely changed her and opened her up to life. In fact, she even met her husband there. I thought maybe that was the answer for me, too. My doctor agreed that it might be good for me. So I quit my job and set off to Hawaii with a friend and all my savings, to visit with the possibility of moving there.

In Hawaii, I became as trim and tan as I'd ever been and fit right in with the bikini scene. This brought men into my life, as well as their expectation of sex, my reluctance, and their demanding, "What's wrong with you?" I couldn't defend myself because I believed they were right, that there was something wrong with me.

One night I met a man in a nightclub who told me that I could find the answer to all my problems with marijuana. I was 21 and had never tried it before. We went to his place. In the darkened living room, we smoked from an elaborate pipe contraption that had colorful tubes undulating around it. I puffed at it as he instructed me to and soon began to feel clouded and paranoid. He had made a remark earlier that I'd look good with a three-inch scar on my cheek, and I started worrying about being there with him. While he was getting me some wine, a glass slipped out of his hand and broke. He put the pieces aside. I remembered his scar remark, and began to get more and more nervous. He started making suggestions that I should feel more loving towards my fellow man, him in particular. I didn't. I felt panicky and feared what he was going to do to me.

I told him I felt dizzy from the pot, and he had me lay down on the floor. As I closed my eyes there was a luminous flash in my head and I could vividly see myself lying there as a skeleton, white glaring bones against a brilliant background of fluorescent red. Had he given me a hallucinogenic? I felt totally out of control. Then I began to feel as if I looked like an ugly old witch with my face full of wrinkles and warts and contorted expressions. I hid my face in my hands and curled up into a ball. This was how I really saw myself and I wanted to hide. He was dancing around me weirdly, saying that he wanted to make love to me. I told him I didn't want to, that I was a virgin. He laughed and said he didn't believe me, but I insisted. He looked at me disdainfully and eventually took me home.

This whole episode had convinced me that I did not fit into this world. Not only was I paranoid, but I was a prude as well. I was angry and frightened of men and only seemed to attract and be attracted to men who were outwardly charming, but inwardly hated women. I saw that I would always be alone, and I'd rather be dead than live my whole life that way. If I couldn't find happiness in a paradise like Hawaii, then where could I find it? Nowhere, was my conclusion. I went shopping and bought bread, butter, a pineapple, and 600 aspirin that were on sale. When I went back home I would wait for the right time to take them.

Once I was home, I hid the aspirins in my dresser drawer and felt relieved to know they were there. I didn't feel so trapped. A few nights after my return from Hawaii, I went to a dance and met someone who was intelligent, fun, handsome, and had his own airplane. We began dating and my hopes were raised. Will he turn my life around? He was gentle with me and wasn't rushing me into sex; I began to fall in love with him.

After a month of dating, his patience began to wear thin, and I reluctantly gave in to my first sexual experience. Under the circumstances, it didn't go well at all. I was angry at him for pressuring me, and he was angry at me. He took me home and I never saw him again. "Everyone I love leaves me," I thought, and old wounds were reopened more painfully than ever before. Everytime I heard an airplane fly over, I wondered if it was him. There were many airplanes that summer and each one deepened the ache. Finally I felt that only 600 aspirins could ease my pain. It was at this point that I took the 80 aspirins and was hospitalized.

I began to see my psychiatrist again, but it didn't help. Two months passed and during that time I drank to try and get high, but now alcohol just deepened my depression. I'd go to dances with friends who were focused on husband-hunting, but I had no interest in that and would go out to the cold, dark car and wait hours for them to come out so that I could go home. I started a new job that was straight typing eight hours a day. I hated it and couldn't bear to go to work. I didn't like living at home, yet I was afraid to go out on my own. My whole life stretched out before me as either an endless, joyless bore, or an agonizing pain. I was only 21 years old, but it felt like my life was over.

I pretended to my doctor that I was feeling better. I told him I was having trouble sleeping and asked for a prescription for sleeping pills. He believed me and gave me a prescription for 25 seconals. I saved them, waiting for the final evidence that would convince me to end it all.

Deadly Serious

One night, I went to the beach where there were nightclubs and arcades and lots of people my age, but it just accentuated my separateness. I ran into a guy I knew from earlier days. He had grown bitter after losing friends in the Vietnam War. He looked at me with disgust and said, "Girls like you (who don't put out) should stay home." "Girls like me, who don't fit in, should give up," I thought. It was the push I needed to give me the courage to finally end it all.

Later that night, when I was alone in my room, I took out the sleeping pills and stared at them. I convinced myself that this was the only way. I felt hopeless. I could not imagine my life ever getting better. I could not imagine being without this constant hurt. Always before my suicide attempts had been chancy, like Russian Roulette, not knowing if the pills I was taking could kill. This time I knew there really was a bullet in the chamber—prescription sleeping pills and alcohol were a lethal combination. I thought of Marilyn Monroe— "Don't be a coward," I prodded myself. "Do it!"

I poured a glass of wine and began to swallow the sleeping pills, hurrying so that I would not change my mind. I was scared. I was crying. I was shaking. But it was too late to back out now. My resolve was strong. Quickly, I drifted off.

The next thing I remember is looking up from what seemed like a deep, dark hole and seeing nurses' faces huddled around me. I was screaming, "Why didn't you let me die?" I was so furious that even in the stupor that enveloped me I could feel my rage. I tried to thrash about, but couldn't move because I was strapped down with IVs in my arms.

When I became more conscious and calmed down, my mother told me that she had gone into my bedroom at noon and found me still in bed. She had tried to wake me, but my breathing was labored and I would not wake up. She immediately called an ambulance which came and rushed me to the emergency ward. I was in a coma for 36 hours. She told me that as I was coming out of the coma, she was embarrassed because I was screaming and sounded like a "spoiled brat." "Not even when I'm unconscious am I allowed to express anger," I thought bitterly.

My mother had been a nurse for several years at the hospital I was in, and just the day before had made a job change to a nearby state mental hospital. Now, barely out of the coma, I was being transferred to that very mental hospital. It was as if I was following her, as if in my anger I was saying to her, "Look what you have done to me!"

From the check-in room at the mental hospital I could hear pounding and obscenities being screamed from locked rooms in all directions. I was put into a large, dorm-like room for women that contained about 30 beds. There was also a day room where everyone spent their time. I saw a girl about my age and noticed how slow and mechanical her movements were as she lifted a cigarette to her mouth and held it poised in mid-air. By the next day, I was moving in just the same manner because I was heavily sedated. Four times a day, a bell would ring for us to stand in line where I received a cup filled with various multi-colored pills (which included Tofranil and Stelezine), and, as the nurses watched, I swallowed them with water.

I felt so numbed that it was difficult to concentrate enough to read. Each day we would rise at 6:00 A.M., sweep the day room, wash the floor, then trudge off to breakfast, ushered by the nurses through a series of locked doors. After breakfast, we all showered together. None of the bathrooms had doors, only curtains. For someone like me, who craved privacy, this place was Hell. Many of the women on my ward were psychotic. One young girl would chase after me, grab my sleeve and wipe her nose on it. Another had had her front teeth taken out because she bit people. Two older ladies continually walked around in circles, one behind the other, never speaking a word. I desperately wanted to get out of that hospital, but 30 days was the customary minimum commitment. Finally, I was interviewed by a group of doctors, and since I wanted out so badly, I said all the right things. After two weeks I was released on an outpatient basis.

Out in the world again, still living at home, I took Triavil four times a day, which was a combination tranquilizer and antidepressant. It was wonderful to no longer feel the constant barbs of anxiety and sadness that had become a way of life for me. But my feelings in general were numbed and the drug made me lethargic, so I ate more and began to put on weight.

A lot of my friends were married now, but marriage for me had always been a vague notion. Although some part of me was always waiting for someone to come and "save me," I didn't really believe that would happen. I was just playing at relationships, only going out with noncommittal men who were like playmates helping me pass the time. One of my boyfriends was a certified psychopath who had been admitted to the same mental hospital that I'd been in.

I wasn't working and I didn't want to. I drank alcohol often, and though I knew that mixing it with the Triavil was dangerous, I didn't care. I had never really thought in terms of a future. My energy had always been mainly focused on my impending death. Life still held no great importance for me, so if I died, I died. I was just marking time at a dead end. But my compulsion towards suicide had lessened because the Triavil numbed the emotional intensity that had fueled my compulsion. Without suicide as an option, however, I needed some direction that would take me beyond this dead end. I began to think about what I'd learned in the "power-of-positive-thinking" books I'd read. I believed that if I could change my negative attitude, my life would change. I read a book on self-hypnosis and for several nights at bedtime I relaxed myself into a receptive state and made suggestions for a better life, asking God for help and guidance. I was praying for my life.

Within a few days, I received an answer. My brother invited me to visit him in Santa Barbara, California, where he was now married and had two beautiful little girls. (I couldn't know then that years later I would end up on a long distance phone call with one of these girls as she overdosed on pills, and that both of them as teenagers would be hospitalized for suicide attempts.) Santa Barbara had a beauty and climate that soothed my nerves and brightened my outlook, so I decided to stay.

I was still on Triavil four times a day, which helped calm me enough to take risks I wouldn't ordinarily have taken. I got an apartment with some other women, got a part-time job, and began attending college. I started going to a psychologist weekly and soon developed a huge crush on him. He was safe, on the other side of a desk, married, and inaccessible.

Week after week I would have his attention as I tried to convince him why I was not fit for this world. At home I fantasized about him rescuing me from a suicide attempt, falling in love with me, and saving me from my sad life. He was usually cool and detached and I wanted to shake him out of that detachment. I wanted him to show me he had feelings, that I wasn't the only one. I wanted him to be real with me, to show me that he cared. One day, I threatened to jump out of his office window, which was several stories up. The alarm on his face gratified me, because I had finally broken through his cool and could see that he cared.

After several months of therapy he felt that the pills I was taking were making it hard for him to get to my feelings, and he tried to talk me into getting off of them. Although the dosage had been gradually lessened, I was afraid that if I gave them up completely, all the painful feelings would come back and swamp me. He kept urging me, until finally I gave up the pills. It was scary as the sensitivity returned, anxiety sharpened, and fears surrounded me; but I knew he was right. It was time to deal with it all. The pills had been helpful in stabilizing me, but now they were preventing me from growing beyond that.

For the first time, I began expressing to him the depths of my feelings, and he responded with caring and concern. I had always thought of myself as weak and cowardly, afraid to face life. But he told me that he thought I was very strong to have endured this long. I had never thought of it that way before and began to feel better about myself. Then, one day I overheard him asking his secretary where my file was, and she, not knowing I was listening, said, "Look in the 'born-to-lose' file." I felt stunned and betrayed. It sounded like an "in" joke. Did they make fun of me? Did he reveal my material? He denied it, but my trust in him was destroyed. "This always happens when I trust and let myself care," I thought to myself. I stopped seeing him shortly after that.

I was on my own again. The bitterness I felt at being betrayed poisoned any positive thoughts I had cultivated. Without the aid of pills and counseling, my unleashed negative feelings began to grow until, eventually, I couldn't stand myself or my life. All I could feel was hate, suspicion, guilt, and fear, and those ugly weeds were clenched around my throat and heart and I was suffocating. I was becoming more and more withdrawn and isolated. I had brick-by-brick erected an impenetrable wall around me, repelling people and discouraging friendships. I was trapped inside, alone. My protective wall had become my prison. I knew I needed help but I couldn't trust or talk to anyone, and I despised myself for the self-pity which infested my life.

I was so sunk in despair that I began to devise my most gruesome and terrifying suicide plan, and I thought about it constantly. I didn't want to be found this time. There was a pile of old tires, brush, and weeds beside my house. I planned to swallow about 100 assorted pills (Tofranil, Stelezine, Triavil) that I'd been hoarding since my hospital days, bury myself under the rubbish and wait to die. I imagined that rats would be crawling around my body, gnawing on it. I was trembling with fear and sadness and anger that my life had come to this. Dying beneath a pile of rubbish would be a statement of how I felt about myself and my life. Could I go through with it? If I didn't, what was the alternative? I refused to go on living in this Hell that my life had become. But if I were to try and climb out of it and back into hope again, I would be so vulnerable should disappointments occur. I was afraid to let myself feel good or care about anything because every time I had in the past I had lost it and been devastated. As it was, I didn't fear disappointment because I was so far down that I didn't have far to fall.

I could feel how attached I was to the thought of suicide. I realized that I was addicted to it and would reach for it like an alcoholic reaches for a drink. It offered me an escape when pressures got too great, or when reality became too unpleasant. It gave me some feeling of control over my life. It had become a part of my identity and my sense of importance. But now this coping mechanism threatened my life, confronting me with rats and rubbish and one hundred brain-numbing pills. A lifetime of half-heartedly playing at life and playing at death, never fully committing to either, had finally culminated in a frustration that now demanded, "Do it or don't do it! Make up your mind!"

A Life Worth Living

I went to bed in the darkness; I prayed to God for a sign that life was worth living. As I was praying, I heard a sound of movement in the room and I froze. I turned on the light and looked in the direction of the movement. A candle I had in a candle holder on the wall had fallen to one side, pointing to the poster that was hanging next to it that said, "GET THY SHIT TOGETHER." I smiled to myself, "Is that you God?" The next day, as I was writing in my diary about what had happened, it happened again! I was getting the message that I wasn't alone. I thought of the other times I had asked God for help and had received it. God was just waiting for me to ask. It took being trapped in the pits of despair with no way out but death before I could turn to God and say, "Help me! I'll do anything you want! Just please help me stop the pain!" If God wanted me to live, then maybe my life had purpose after all. Maybe the alternative to suicide was surrendering to God and trusting that I'd be guided out of the suffering.

From my reading and my experience with self-hypnosis and positive thinking, I knew that if I wanted something strongly enough I could have it, through choosing, visualizing, and focusing my energy on it. Ever since I was a little girl, I'd chosen to think negatively in order to protect myself from disappointment. Because that's what I had focused on, that's what I got. Negativity became a habit that became a way of life. If I were to choose life, I would have to deliberately change my focus and my thoughts and create a new habit of positiveness.

The possibility of becoming committed to living was starting to do equal battle with the wish to die. As I'd once gathered evidence for why I should die, I now began to gather evidence for why I should live. I remembered what my doctor had said about me being strong. Maybe I was strong enough to turn my life around and heal myself.

One grand gesture towards life would be to quit smoking. I felt that if I could do that, I could do anything. I used self-hypnosis and strongly suggested that I would "effortlessly stop smoking." I did this for three nights and quit cold turkey (and have not smoked since). This was such a powerful statement to me that it created a ripple effect, and I began to exercise and eat more nutritiously. The more healthy I felt, the more healthy I wanted to feel. It was exciting to experience that I could have some kind of control over changing my life, and I began to believe that I really could heal myself. Finally, at age 25, I made the decision to commit to life.

Once I made up my mind there was no turning back. I directed all my energy towards good health, learning ways to relax, and developing positive coping mechanisms. The first and most important thing I did was to meditate twice a day, and I immediately began to feel more relaxed and clear. I also eliminated things from my diet that contributed to tension, like salt, sugar, alcohol, and caffeine. I began to exercise regularly, and I felt even better.

It wasn't always an easy time for me though. There were many ups and downs, and I sometimes felt like I was trying to walk with a frightened child wrapped around my leg. Many mornings I woke up with a habitual feeling of boredom, fear, and dread of what the day held. But when I recognized that as a habit-feeling, I'd remind myself, "Choose how you want to feel." I then deliberately created a good feeling by thinking about what was positive about the day, and soon I had developed a new habit of waking up feeling happy.

One of the most freeing things I have learned is that I'm not a helpless victim buffeted about by unlucky circumstances. I have become more and more empowered by the realization that my attitude creates my experience. When I was stuck in my negativity, all I could see was negativity, and I would only let in what confirmed my feeling that the world was a bad place. I couldn't see all the good that was offered me, and I couldn't feel the love of family and friends that had been there all along.

I've stopped being angry at my mother, and this has allowed me to experience all the good things about her that I wouldn't let myself see before. I let go of my resentment towards her when I became aware that it was my hanging onto it that was causing my pain. I needed to change my attitude towards her and forgive her. So, at the end of my meditations I began to visualize my mother smiling at me. At first it was difficult, but each time I persisted until I was able to see and feel it. Then I visualized us hugging, apologizing to one another, and forgiving each other. Eventually, I could feel my heart open to her. I wrote her a loving letter, telling her what I appreciated about her, because now that I'd freed myself from that rigid image I'd held of her I could see her many good qualities and could understand that she'd always sincerely tried to do the best she could. Once I was able to feel loving towards her, it allowed her to be more loving towards me. It was like getting a new mother. I did the same forgiveness process with the other members of my family.

I know now that I am the one who gets to choose how I feel. I get to choose to hang on to old hurts or to let them go, to feel good, or to feel bad. No one can "make" me feel a certain way — it is my reaction that causes me pain. I can't control how other people are towards me, but I can control my reaction to them.

Having a positive attitude was tremendously helpful, but I found that it sometimes was not enough. When feelings were not acknowledged and attended to, they would sneak up on me and bash me with a club to get my attention. I needed to learn how to process them constructively. I began to attend a peer-counseling therapy class (which I was in for four years), where we learned counseling techniques that helped us evoke in each other emotional release, and we learned to facilitate understanding the origin of the pain. I was no longer a helpless patient, but the therapist as well. As I learned this new skill, I gained more confidence in my ability to help myself and others.

In this group we were encouraged and praised for expressing emotions. They were no longer treated like thorny little monsters that had to be hid away in a closet. They were now paraded out for all to see and applaud. To see that others had the same feelings that I had, and to experience them in a safe, supportive group, was a huge healing for me. I realized that the intensity of my feelings, which had always made me feel that I was worse than everyone else, was in truth a natural consequence of feelings being repressed and needing some kind of outlet. Some people develop diseases. Some create dramas and accidents. Some people turn it in on themselves and become depressed and suicidal.

The life force demands expression one way or another. The imploded energy of my denied inner self would finally burst into an explosion that demanded, "I'm alive! I exist! I'm here!" My suicide attempts were, in effect, life attempts. Although one of my acts of self-destruction could have killed me, eventually, because of the imminent danger involved, they gave me the impetus I needed to commit to life.

I realize now that resisting my feelings is what caused far more pain than the feelings themselves. As I allow my feelings to flow, they're like little rain bursts or thunderstorms that pass through and are gone. They no longer build into life-threatening hurricanes. The more I feel my feelings, the more connected I am with life and with myself. Sometimes during these years of recovery I've experienced deep pain, but with suicide no longer an option, I could only surrender to the pain and ride it out, praying to God that if I must suffer at least let me grow from it. Once I allow the process and stop resisting, I'm always brought to understanding, growth, and healing.

I awoke from a dream not long ago with these words sounding in my head, "All you have to do in your entire life is to love yourself. That's what you're here for." The more I'm able to accept my feelings and appreciate them as the rich, vibrant colors of my being, the more I'm able to love myself. And once I could feel more loving towards myself, I was able to feel more loving towards others.

Something that has helped me a great deal in healing my fear of intimacy and opening my heart to people is the Intuitive Massage that I practice. It is a slow, nurturing touch that allows me to relate to another in a clear and loving way. It helps me remember and feel compassion for that vulnerable and innocent part of ourselves that longs to be loved and acknowledged just for being who we are.

It was hard to believe back when I was immersed in pain and isolation that life would ever be worth living. But now, still living in Santa Barbara, I sometimes feel like I'm in paradise. I have a strong support system of friends and loved ones, and I continue to be committed to my personal growth process. My sensitivity that had been such a source of pain to me, now serves me in my work as an artist, as a massage technician, and in the peer counseling that I do. I've had more relationships with men and I learn and grow from each one. It has never been a strong desire of mine to be married or have children; I now enjoy and feel fulfilled in my single lifestyle. My most important relationship is with myself and with God, and because of that I seldom feel alone anymore.

I've learned recently that two years ago my high school friend Helen finally put a gun to her head and killed herself. I wish I could have talked to her and told her that there really is a way out of despair. Fortunately, I was able to convince my niece of that during her phone call to me. I believe she had called me because she was reaching out for help. After she had swallowed 50 Tylenol, she told me, "I'm beginning to get a headache."

"Take a Tylenol," I joked, and she laughed.

"See, if you can laugh, then it can't be all bad," I told her. The humor had eased the tension somewhat, and finally she began to tell me what was bothering her. She'd had an argument with her father and felt that he didn't love her. She was hurt and angry, and she didn't know how else to express it, just as I hadn't when I was her age. Overdosing on pills was a dramatic way of saying, "I hurt! I'm angry!" I told her, "You're taking it out on yourself. Don't hurt yourself. You don't deserve that. Go and talk to your dad. Tell him how you're feeling."

But she was afraid to tell him, as I'd been afraid to tell my mother. She got him to the phone, and I told him what she had done.

"Oh my God!" he gasped, and I learned later, he threw his arms around her and hugged her tightly and cried, "Why do you want to die! Don't you know how much I love you?" This is what she had wanted—to know that her life mattered to someone, and to feel that she was loved. That is what I'd wanted, too, but I was unable to feel loved until I could love myself. Now, after all these years, I do.

Resources

Alcohol and Drug Abuse

Alateen, Al-Anon Family Group
Headquarters, Inc.
P.O. Box 182
Madison Square Station
New York, NY 10159
(212) 683-1771

Alcoholics Anonymous
General Service Office
P.O. Box 459
Grand Central Station
New York, NY 10163
(212) 686-1100

American Council for Drug Education
5820 Hubbard Drive
Rockville, MD 20852
(301) 984-5700

American Medical Society on Alcoholism
12 West 21st Street, 7th floor
New York, NY 10010
(212) 206-6770

Association of Halfway House
Alcoholism Programs of North America
786 East 7th Street
St. Paul, MN 55106
(612) 771-0933

Children of Alcoholics Foundation, Inc.
540 Madison Avenue, 23rd floor
New York, NY 10022
(212) 980-5860

COCAINE ANONYMOUS
P.O. Box 1367
Culver City, CA 90232
(213) 839-1141

COCANON Family Groups
Box 3969
Hollywood, CA 90028
(213) 859-2206

Drug Enforcement Administration
Public Affairs Office
1405 I Street, NW
Washington, DC 20537
(202) 633-1469

Hazelden Foundation
Box 11
Center City, MN 55012
(800) 328-9000

Drugs Anonymous
P.O. Box 473
Ansonia Station
New York, NY 10023
(212) 874-0700

Mothers Against Drunk Driving
669 Airport Freeway #310
Hurst, TX 76053
(817) 268-6233

Naranon (family support)
350 West 5th Street - Suite 207
San Pedro, CA 90731

Narcotics Anonymous
P.O. Box 9999
Van Nuys, CA 91409
Hotline: (818) 997-3822
World Service Office: (818) 780-3951

National Association of Alcoholism and
Drug Abuse Counselors, Inc.
951 South George Mason Drive #204
Arlington, VA 22204
(703) 920-4644

National Association of Alcoholism
Treatment Programs, Inc.
2082 Michelson Drive
Irvine, CA 92715
(714) 476-8204

National Center for Alcohol Education
(NCAE)
1601 North Kent Street
Arlington, VA 22209

National Clearinghouse for Alcohol Information
P.O. Box 2345
Rockville, MD 20852
(301) 468-2600

National Clearinghouse for Alcohol Information
P.O. Box 2345
Rockville, MD 20852
(301) 468-2600

National Clearinghouse for Drug Abuse Information
P.O. Box 416
Kensington, MD 20795
(800) 638-2045

National Institute on Alcohol Abuse
Parklawn Building
5600 Fishers Lane
Rockville, MD 20852
(301) 443-3885

Parents' Resource Institute for Drug Education (PRIDE)
100 Edgewood Avenue - Suite 1216
Atlanta, GA 30303
(800) 241-7946

Eating Disorders

American Association of Eating Disorders Counselors
2324 South Coast Highway
Laguna Beach, CA 92651
(714) 494-8227

Anorexia, Bulimia Care, Inc.
P.O. Box 213
Lincoln Center, MA 01773
(617) 259-9767

Anorexia Nervosa and Related Eating Disorders
P.O. Box 5102
Eugene, OR 97405
(503) 344-1144

American Anorexia/Bulimia Assoc.
133 Cedar Lane
Teaneck, NJ 07666
(201) 836-1800

The Bridge/National Anorexic Aid Society
4897 Karl Road
Columbus, OH 43229
(614) 486-2833

Cigarette Smoking

American Heart Association
7320 Greenville Avenue
Dallas, TX 75231
(214) 373-6300

American Lung Association
1740 Broadway
New York, NY 10019
(212) 245-8000

The StopSmoking System
National Heart, Lung and Blood Institute
Department of Health and Human Services
13201 Glen Road
Gaithersburg, MD 20760
(301) 496-5166

Suicide

International Association for Suicide Prevention
Suicide Prevention and Crisis Center
1811 Trusdale Drive
Burlingame, CA 94010
(415) 877-5604

National Save-a-Life League
4520 4th Avenue - Suite MH3
New York, NY 11220
(212) 492-4067

Parents of Suicides
c/o Bergen-Passaic T.C.F.
P.O. Box 373
Inglewood, NJ 07631
(201) 894-0042

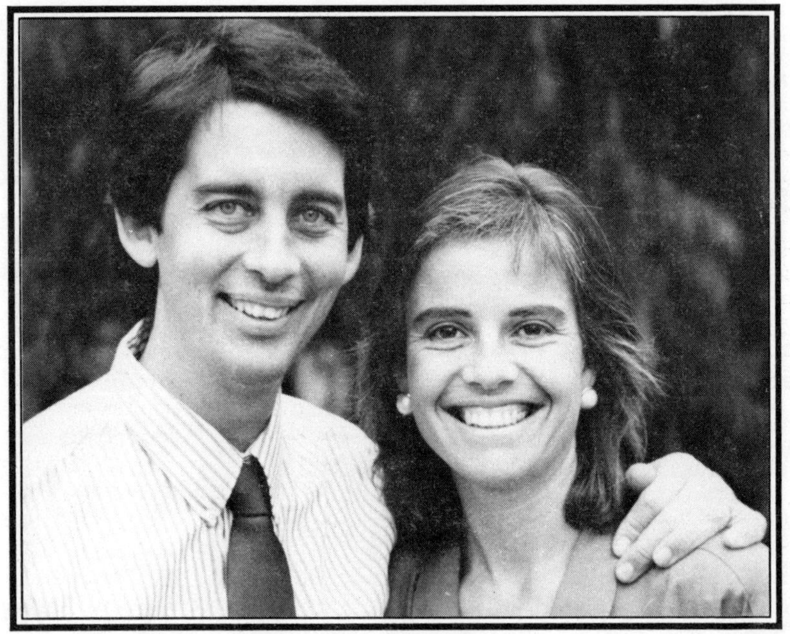

Leigh Cohn and Lindsey Hall

About the Editors

When Lindsey Hall and her husband, Leigh Cohn wrote *Eat Without Fear* as a booklet in 1980, it was the first publication solely about bulimia. They followed with two additional booklets on this subject and later included them all in the book, *BULIMIA: A Guide to Recovery*. Their works have been used in thousands of colleges, high schools, hospitals, and by professional therapists throughout the world. They have taught courses about eating disorders in more than 20 colleges and universities, and they have conducted workshops on overcoming bulimia. Lindsey was the first bulimic to appear on national television. Leigh has had more than 50 articles on this subject published in newspapers and magazines throughout the United States, and has written books in other areas, as well.

Lindsey graduated from Stanford University with a degree in Psychology, and Leigh earned a M.A.T. in English Education from Northwestern University. They established "The Eating Disorders Bookshelf Catalogue" which included the most comprehensive selection of materials in that field. Prior to the publication of *Recoveries,* they renamed their catalogue "The Gürze Bookshelf Catalogue" and expanded with titles on alcoholism, drug abuse, co-dependency, adult children of alcoholics, and the nature of addiction. In addition to editing *Recoveries,* they are writing more books and are both active in health education and publishing.

Lindsey and Leigh enjoy working together and have a happy, loving marriage. They are the proud parents of two sons, Neil and Charlie. They feel fortunate that their projects have helped others to become happier and more self-fulfilled.